PRAISE FOR *OH BABY!*

Maria has a way of telling it like it is from a very personal perspective. While she shares her own motherhood experiences, most will be completely relatable to new and nervous moms looking for some reassurance that everything is okay. Readers will find it easy to flip to their current concern as the chapters are laid out in a succinct, easy-to-read format. A sort of up-to-date *What to Expect*, readers will also learn what to **accept**.

—Kathy Buckworth, author of *I Am So the Boss of You*

Advice you want in a tone you'll love. Lianos-Carbone mixes the facts and support every new parent needs with the smile-at-the-whole-crazy-ride we want in that moment. No patronizing help here; she tells us exactly what to expect and—even better—reminds us that new parenting is worth the struggle.

—Deborah Gilboa, MD, author of *Get the Behavior You Want . . . Without Being the Parent You Hate!*

If *Oh Baby! A Mom's Self-Care Survival Guide for the First Year* had been around when I had my first baby, the transition might have been a whole lot different! Must-read for every new mom.

—Natalie Klein, CEO of Hot Moms Club

When I gave birth to my first child in 1980, I wondered what was wrong with me when reality didn't match my idealized vision of blissful motherhood. *Oh Baby!* would have saved me a lot of anxiety. Maria writes like a big sister, or a best girlfriend who had a baby before you, sharing secrets of the motherhood trade in an intelligent, down-to-earth manner. Doctors should hand this book to all their expectant moms.

—Mary Potter Kenyon, mother of eight, author or coauthor of six books, including *Mary & Me: A Lasting Link through Ink* and the award-winning *Refined by Fire: A Journey of Grief and Grace*

Funny, thoughtful, and non-judgmental, *Oh Baby! A Mom's Self-Care Survival Guide for the First Year* is the coffee chat with a friend (in book form) that every new mother needs. Maria Lianos-Carbone presents the big and small challenges of motherhood in a supportive and honest light. The easy-to-read format of the chapters are filled with practical tips, real mom experiences, and milestones for moms and babies alike. Oh Baby! is a great companion on your journey through motherhood.

—Caroline Fernandez, owner of ParentClub.ca and author of *Boredom Busters* and *More Boredom Busters*

Written after both personal experience and research about best practices, Maria offers an incredibly detailed approach for moms, in particular, after the birth of their baby. While *Oh Baby!* offers a great deal of information about what to expect from baby, a theme that flows throughout encourages new moms to take care of their own needs too–an important message, I believe. This book is easy to read and relatable, offers humour, and has great illustrations. The mom-to-mom sections are a welcome addition too.

—Sara Dimerman, psychologist and author of *Am I a Normal Parent* and *How to Influence Your Kids for Good*

In my first year of pregnancy, I have turned to Maria in moments of worry and fear, many times over. As a dear friend and an experienced mother who is deeply connected to raising children, and has a strong and progressive outlook on bringing up babies, Maria was able to guide me out of any panic. Maria has taken her knowledge and experience and turned it into a book, available to anyone. *Oh Baby!* is filled with funny anecdotes and sensible information backed by research in an easy-to-understand format.

Would make a fantastic baby shower gift!

—Anita Doron, filmmaker (*The Lesser Blessed*), screenwriter (*The Breadwinner*), and TED Fellow

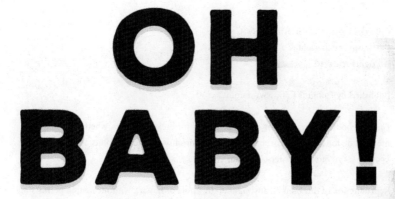

OH BABY!

FAMILIUS

Published by Familius LLC, www.familius.com

Familius books are available at special discounts for bulk purchases, whether for sales pro-
motions or for family or corporate use. For more information, contact Familius Sales at
559-876-2170 or email orders@familius.com.

Library of Congress Cataloging-in-Publication Data
2017958503

Print ISBN 9781945547706
Ebook ISBN 9781641700061

Printed in the United States of America

Edited by Michele Robbins
Cover design by David Miles
Book design by Brooke Jorden

10 9 8 7 6 5 4 3 2 1

First Edition

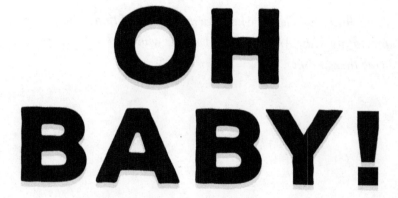

OH BABY!

A Mom's Self-Care Survival Guide for the First Year

MARIA LIANOS-CARBONE

To my husband, Genio, who gave me the gift of time to write, and to my kids, Anthony and Daniel, who gave me the gift of being their mother.

CONTENTS

INTRODUCTION

When you become pregnant, you think you do a great job preparing for baby to arrive. You buy all of baby's essentials, baby-proof the home, and have the car seat and stroller ready. The nursery is painted, furniture is assembled, and clothes are washed and put away.

I had taken birth classes, toured the maternity ward, and read every book there was. I was so ready! But then labor and delivery completely threw off everything I prepared for. Baby was born, and then I realized I had NO idea what I was doing. I thought it would be a piece of cake to feed the baby, change his diaper, and have him fall asleep. What was I thinking?!

Nothing quite prepares you for motherhood. While you may think you have all the bases covered in time for baby's arrival, you may not be mentally and emotionally prepared for the changes you'll experience as a new mother. Oh baby! But what about Mom?

Motherhood changes you fundamentally as a human being and as a woman. It forces you to question everything about yourself—your instincts, your core values, and your goals. Motherhood also challenges you in every respect: your decision-making, patience, and strength of character.

When I had my first son, I thought that some moms always looked like they had it together. Motherhood seemed to come so naturally to them. I'd wonder: *Are they really enjoying motherhood like they appear to be?*

After some prodding, these women started to magically open up. Like an epiphany, we seemed to suddenly realize that we were all struggling to cope with the challenges of motherhood. Why were we so afraid to talk about it?

Part of it was cultural—we were "supposed" to know how to be a mom, just like our moms. We were supposed to be able to do it all—and do it all with a smile. Part of it was womanly instinct—we were supposed to be natural at breastfeeding, changing diapers, and dealing with screaming babies.

Part of what keeps us from really sharing is fear of comparing—we don't want our friends to think that we are having a tough time while they are in complete bliss. Part of it is fear of failure—we don't want to fail at being a mom. We must figure this out!

The truth is, motherhood is the most challenging yet rewarding lifetime experience many of us will ever have. Through my journey into motherhood, I have learned many valuable lessons that have helped me to grow into the person that I am and always wanted to be.

When baby is born, the focus shifts to him. Baby books on how to parent baby are abundant. But what about how Mom is feeling? This book will focus on Mom and how she can survive that challenging yet joyful first year with baby.

A Letter to My Newborn Baby

Dear baby boy,

I'm so happy that you're here in my arms. I've been waiting for this day to come, and now it's finally here. And it's so much more than I ever imagined.

Holding you in my arms is something I dreamed of for so long. I could picture it in my mind, and it's the best feeling in the world. I'm so lucky that I'm your mom.

I felt like I was missing something my entire life, and now I know why—I was waiting for you. I've loved you since I first learned you were growing in my belly, and I will love you more and more every day as you grow. I'll be here to nurture you and give you the best life I can possibly give.

Please know that I will do my very best to guide you and protect you. Even if I make mistakes, and I know I will, please know that I will always love you with all of my heart. I hope to be the mommy that you deserve.

I hope I can guide you to be a kind, loving, and sweet little boy who cares about other people and loves ever so deeply. I hope you grow up to fulfill wonderful dreams and live a life that is full of joy and adventure.

I worry, though, because although I'm here to protect you now, once you're older, you will learn about sadness too. The world is not always safe and kind. But I hope you will continue to see the good in people and the miracles of life, as I do in you.

Thank you for bringing such love and peace to my heart and my soul.

Love,
Mommy

Chapter One

BRINGING BABY HOME CAN BE DAUNTING

Congratulations! You survived your pregnancy, labor, and delivery! Feelings of joy, love, and happiness consume you and your partner as you welcome your baby into this world. Your family has grown and blossomed, and soon enough, you won't be able to imagine your life before your new bundle of joy arrived.

That long-awaited moment is finally here—it's time to bring baby home and begin your life as a family! It's completely normal to feel as if the entire pregnancy and birth was surreal. Did it actually happen?! Your baby is proof that this all isn't a dream. Despite reading all the pregnancy books, asking your doctor a million questions, and perusing baby blogs, nothing can really prepare you for how you're going to feel when baby arrives.

You and your partner are about to experience a new world of emotions in this chapter of your lives together. You may be feeling a mixture of joy, excitement, and nervousness too. You may FREAK OUT! Yes—while you're happy to bring baby home, you may begin to feel overwhelmed about caring for your newborn baby once you leave the hospital. Knowing that you won't have the guidance of hospital nurses or doctors as you begin the journey of caring for your baby on your own can cause feelings of anxiety. While you're thrilled to bring baby home, you're also super nervous! These conflicting feelings are completely normal and may last a short time while you settle in.

Though you may have some worries as you begin this new adventure, keep things in perspective. For me, it felt so bizarre that I was actually a mother and my husband was a father! We had a moment of disbelief when we looked at each other in our new minivan (yes, it comes with the territory) on our way home from the hospital, and we started giggling like schoolchildren.

This is a special time for you and your partner as you begin this exciting stage of life as a family. Share your concerns, thoughts, and emotions with one another. Be understanding and patient, as your partner may be having feelings very unlike yours. Remember that the more you listen and discuss feelings early on, the less likely hurt feelings and frustrations will develop. Open communication and empathy is crucial to your marriage now more than ever. The natural bonding of parenthood can bring your relationship even closer.

Mom Has Needs, Too!

The first few weeks at home with your new baby can be a challenging time. You may try to keep the same feeding, sleeping, and self-care routine which started during your hospital stay. Keep in mind that newborns cannot tell time, and they don't understand night is for sleeping. Some new moms say these first weeks are the toughest, while for others, the newborn stage is a breeze. Much of this depends on your labor and delivery and your recovery. It helps if you take the time to heal and bond with baby. You'll find you'll naturally move into somewhat of a schedule after the first three months. For now, the focus is to recover and spend time with your sweet little angel.

One of the biggest traps moms fall into is focusing so much time and energy on baby that we forget moms have needs too. When we're so consumed with what baby needs, we forget what WE need. People will tell you that you'll need to rest, but they don't tell you about all the other things that you'll need. Who knew you needed a stool softener or hemorrhoid cream?! (Because that first bowel movement is going to hurt!) From a healthy supply of sanitary pads to stocking up on your favorite morning tea, you will be glad you are prepared.

Every woman's birthing experience is different, so there isn't one specific checklist of things mom will need after giving birth. You may have a fairly easy labor and delivery and a normal recovery, or you may have a long, difficult one requiring an epidural, episiotomy, and antibiotics. You may end up having a scheduled or unscheduled C-section.

Here is a list of things that are helpful to have on hand after you come home. Some of these items will be provided to you at the hospital.

Mom Essentials

- **Your favorite snacks**—you'll be hungry!
- **A cozy bathrobe, pajamas, and slippers.**
- **Comfortable pillows and blankets.**
- **Magazines, books, and a notebook or journal** for recording baby's sleep, feedings, and wet diapers.
- **Camera or smartphone, with charger,** for capturing those first days at home.

- **Baby/parenting reference books.**
- **Bags of frozen peas.** Yes, really! Or an ice pack for sitting during that painful first postpartum week, if you've torn your perineum or had an episiotomy.
- **Bum cushion.** Even for moms who are lucky enough to avoid hemorrhoids, a donut cushion will help make sitting after a C-section, an episiotomy, or tearing much more comfortable.
- **Extra-large underwear.** If you can take a few disposable undies from the hospital, do it! Or buy a few full-brief grandma panties to have at home that you can just throw away. A thong just won't cut it!
- **Maxi pads.** Many women aren't prepared for the amount of lochia—postpartum vaginal discharge, containing blood, mucus, and placental tissue—that is released postpartum. You'll need the huge, super-absorbent kind for the first few days, and as the bleeding tapers off, you may be able to switch to a thinner but still absorbent pad for several weeks. No tampons allowed!
- **Stool softener.** The hospital will give you a stool softener to help with that first bowel movement. But if you are prone to getting constipated, it may be helpful to have a stool softener on hand at home.
- **Sitz bath.** You may receive one of these at the hospital to take home with you. It's like an insert for the toilet that you can fill with warm water to soothe your sore private area. You'll also probably receive a squirt bottle to take home; warm water will definitely be more soothing to clean with after a bathroom call than toilet paper.
- **Hemorrhoid wipes and cream (just in case).** It is very common for women to get hemorrhoids from all the pushing during labor. If you do get hemorrhoids, they will itch and burn. You'll likely receive Tucks from the

hospital, which are witch hazel–soaked pads that will help soothe your privates, but you may need to purchase more.

- **Cabbage.** Whether you're breastfeeding or not, a cool cabbage leaf in your bra helps sooth sore, engorged breasts.
- **Nipple cream.** If breastfeeding, you'll need a good nipple cream as your nipples will be sore at first (see Chapter Four). Check with your doctor or hospital for a baby-safe ointment. You may receive some samples at the hospital, but make sure you have some on hand at home.
- **Nursing bra.** Even if you're not nursing, your breasts will probably feel uncomfortable, as they will be engorged. Since your size may change when your milk comes in, it is a good idea to have a couple of nursing bras to start with.
- **Nursing pads.** Your breasts will leak as they become engorged. You can choose either disposable or reusable/washable pads to keep in your bra.
- **Nursing pillow.** A good nursing pillow isn't just for baby's comfort but also for Mom's. It allows you to sit up straight and brings baby to your breast so you don't slump to bring breast to baby or end up with tired muscles from holding baby in position.
- **Acetaminophen or ibuprofen.** You'll likely receive pain medication from the hospital, but you may need a supply at home. These are both safe for perineal pain after childbirth. Consult your doctor for dosage and any concerns.

In addition to basic mom supplies, you may want to create a baby station in the area of the house where you'll likely spend the most time. For me, this was the main floor of the house in our family room; I created an area set up with a basket of baby essentials so I wouldn't always have to run upstairs to the nursery to change a diaper, wipe a chin, or grab a pacifier. Especially during your recovery period (and later when you're just feeling lazy), having items nearby will help tremendously.

You can even stash a book or two in the baby station. When you're recovering from labor, having a few good parenting books at arm's reach can be helpful. You will be referencing books often . . . several times a day, especially the first year! The more information you're armed with, the more equipped and prepared you'll feel. Some of my favorites were:

- *The Happiest Baby on the Block* by Harvey Karp, MD
- *The Baby Book* by William Sears, MD; Martha Sears, RN; Robert Sears, MD; and James Sears, MD
- *The No-Cry Sleep Solution* by Elizabeth Pantley
- *Your Baby & Child* by Penelope Leach
- *Brain Rules for Baby* by John Medina
- *What to Expect the First Year* (Third Edition) by Heidi Murkoff and Sharon Mazel
- *The Fussy Baby Book* by William and Martha Sears

How You May Be Feeling

Becoming a parent doesn't automatically infuse your brain with everything you need to know to be a good parent. Just because you read about how to diaper, swaddle, or bathe a baby doesn't mean that you'll remember all the steps when actually doing them! It's quite common for new moms to feel uncoordinated and unconfident about taking care of baby. You may feel like you have two left hands. I kept referring to *What to Expect When You're Expecting* to make sure I was swaddling the baby properly even though I had read the book a thousand times! Being a mom is like most things—it requires good training and practice.

I remember first feeling a sense of relief finally being home from the hospital; the four days we spent there felt like an eternity.

But once we were settled in the comfort of our home, the feelings of anxiety kicked in as I realized—*It's just me and the baby.*

If you're like me, you might envision something scary happening to the baby, especially during the night. The first night home, I repeatedly checked to make sure my baby boy was breathing. I had read some terrifying stories and worried myself into extreme unnecessary panic.

That panic can continue throughout the day too. It's completely normal to freak out a little when you realize that you're responsible for keeping this little human being ALIVE. *Oh my goodness, I have to take care of this adorable, beautiful, tiny baby! Am I changing his diaper right? Does he have enough wet diapers? Is he latching properly?*

The constant worry can be overwhelming. This is the time when your partner, family member, or friend can help guide you through your feelings. Your mom, sister, or best friend is just a phone call away; reach out for guidance, for help, or even just to hear a friendly voice. The first week home especially is a time to ask for help. Don't overdo it, even if you think you're ready to bounce back. I know firsthand that for people who are constantly on the go, it's difficult to hang out on a couch or bed. You may feel like you need to be doing more—but you shouldn't.

Whether you are feeling nervous, overwhelmed, or just plain stir crazy, remember that this is very normal. You are not alone. Bringing baby home is an emotional adventure. Be sure to talk to your partner, friend, family, and doctor about your feelings and get help when you need it. (More on this in Chapter Nine.)

Sleep and Rest

These first few weeks are so important for mom and baby. It's important to remember this time is for you to bond with baby and recover. Your partner or family and friends can run errands for you while you rest. I made the terrible mistake of going out on day three of being home and doing some grocery shopping at the local supermarket. I *thought* I was feeling fine, but halfway through my visit, I realized I was very sore down there. I had pushed myself too far. I managed to get home, but I notably experienced a setback in my recovery. Who did I think I was—Superwoman?! I should have stayed home and sent someone else rather than thinking I could do it. If I needed fresh air, I could've just gone outside the house for a few minutes.

You may feel like the four walls are closing in on you, or you may get a touch of cabin fever. Once hubby is off to work and it's just you and the baby, the feeling kicks in that you can't dash out to pick up groceries or grab a coffee. Most of your day will be spent feeding, changing, and holding your baby. Remember: you just went through labor, and it is called "labor" for a reason. Now is the time to take it easy and allow your body time to heal.

If your partner is able to take time off work to stay with you the first week or two, this will help ease the transition. Otherwise, a family member such as your mom, sister, or friend can perhaps offer help. Now is not the time to be a martyr; you're not meant to do this all on your own. It really does take a village!

Sleep When the Baby Sleeps

You may say, *Yeah, right! I've heard that lie before.* While it may be tempting to watch your exquisite baby's face while he sleeps, you should be taking a nap too. I know; you don't want to miss staring at those beautiful little lashes, the pursed lips, and that cute button nose, but it's so important for moms to nap during the day when the baby is sleeping. The biggest hurdle for new parents is sleep deprivation; you will miss those seven hours of straight sleep during the night for many, many months. Not having enough sleep means you won't be able to function normally during the day. Days roll into nights, and with the lack of proper sleep, everything will seem like a big blur.

This is the time when you need rest. The physical recovery from giving birth, along with sleep deprivation, can take a huge toll. After going through the exhausting experience of childbirth, new moms need time to recover. It's important to eat well, drink plenty of fluids, and rest.

If I had it to do all over again, I would take more naps during the day. I could never get enough sleep during the night because the baby would wake two to three times. To prepare for the night-time wakings, even if you can't nap, lie down and rest. Whether relaxing for you means watching TV, listening to music, or reading a book, do whatever it is that helps you feel rested when the baby wakes up. Afternoon naps—followed by a cup of coffee—were the only way I could function the remainder of the day!

Can I Get Anything Done?

Nurturing a newborn takes up most of your day. You may think you can cook a lovely dinner for you and your partner to enjoy after a long day, but in reality, you're lucky if you've managed to brush your teeth!

It's a healthy and helpful realization to accept the fact that the house will be messier. It's okay! It's alright that the sink is full of dishes, the bed isn't made, and the laundry is piling up. You won't be able to dedicate two straight hours to cleaning when you have an infant to care for. Instead, do one load of laundry or a few dishes at a time. Breaking up what seems to feel like huge projects into smaller tasks can help you overcome feeling overwhelmed. The household chores can wait; they will always be there (unfortunately).

You also may be surprised by how much time you spend breastfeeding. I didn't know that I'd be basically stuck on the couch or bed with my breasts hanging out, teaching my little one to suck. It really helps to understand that breastfeeding is work too. Give yourself credit as you devote a large part of your day to breastfeeding and accept that other things will take a back-burner position for a while.

The little things you didn't notice before will be a delight now. You'll come to realize how much you appreciate your first cup of coffee or having a few minutes to take a hot shower. Cherish the few moments you have to yourself, because you won't have many of them!

Your day may look a little like this:

1. Wake up and have a sip of coffee.
2. Nurse/feed baby.
3. Burp baby.
4. Change baby's diaper.
5. Change baby's diaper again after a blowout.
6. Warm up coffee in microwave.
7. Baby sleeps. (And Mom rests too!)
8. Change baby's diaper.
9. Nurse/feed baby.
10. Burp baby.
11. Warm up coffee in microwave.

It Does Get Easier

Everything will become easier with time. At first, changing your newborn's diaper may seem daunting. Feeding and burping baby may seem like an Olympic sport. You and your baby are getting to know each other, and you and your partner are adjusting to your new roles as a family unit.

But things will get easier! Hold on to the thought that right around that six-week mark, you'll start to get into a groove. With time and practice, you will become calmer and more confident; you'll be able to change a diaper with your eyes closed. And since your body has had time to heal, you will be amazed at how much better you feel. Most soreness should be gone, and you will likely feel great to have your body back (well, for the most part). More about that in Chapter Seventeen.

After the challenges you've encountered during the newborn phase, you will soon be rewarded with one of the most gratifying milestones when your little angel looks up and throws you a genuine smile. That one simple expression will make the sleepless nights, the diaper explosions, and the leaking breasts you've endured worth every second.

Chapter Two

ARE VISITORS WELCOME—OR NOT?

A new baby causes huge excitement within the family circle. Family members, friends, neighbors, and co-workers will all want to schedule a time to visit your new bundle of joy. The visitors will want to come in droves! They may innocently forget that you're recovering from any kind of birth trauma—it's now all about the baby. Who can blame them for wanting to meet the new addition to the family, your mini-me?

While it's a wonderful gesture, and only natural, you'll need to discuss the "rules" with your partner *before* the entire army of cousins arrives at your doorstep. Communicate with your partner and your family about visitors ahead of time, and let them know your wishes well in advance—ideally weeks before baby's birth. Depending on how difficult your childbirth was, you may wish to have visitors right away—or not!

You may change your mind once you realize how tired you'll be or how overwhelmed you may feel. On the flip side, you might feel that you're up to having visitors and welcome having family over to keep you company. Either way, listen to yourself and don't be afraid to express your wishes.

Now, if you already know that your mother-in-law or Aunt Bessie is going to be camping outside your hospital room or your front door, you'll need to have laid out the groundwork *early on*. If it's a relative on hubby's side, have him deal. Otherwise, let your relatives know well in advance that you don't expect a visit until week two.

If You're Not Open to Visitors Right Away

For some, breastfeeding is a huge learning curve not just the first few days but for several weeks. I know I wasn't hugely comfortable popping out my breast to nurse a poorly latching infant in front of my uncle! No, I enjoyed my privacy, thank you very much. I wanted the privacy for everything to sink in because I JUST HAD A BABY. My husband became a DAD. We wanted to cherish these precious moments on our own, before all the craziness of our family and friends descended upon us.

If friends or relatives are inviting themselves over to see the baby and you're not up for company or you know they will out-stay their welcome, don't be afraid to turn them down gently. If you've always been accommodating and shy, especially with your partner's family, you need to set boundaries now more than ever.

This time is for you to rest, recover, and become comfortable with your baby. You're in no condition or mood to entertain family who are not there to pitch in but rather create more work or stress for you. There's no point in having *My Big Fat Greek Wedding* arrive at your doorstep unless they're willing to help cook a meal, drop off food, or watch the baby so you can have a shower. Otherwise, their presence might make you feel frustrated.

Also, you're not obligated to host anyone. A visit means your guests can help themselves to the coffee machine or a glass of water. Don't feel like you need to entertain guests as you normally would by serving finger foods, snacks, or coffee and dessert. There will be time for that later on; right now, it's all about congratulating you and your spouse and meeting your new bundle of joy.

Out-of-Town Guests

If your parents or in-laws are from out of town, you will have to decide whether you and your partner will welcome them to stay with you when baby arrives. If it's the first grandchild, everyone will be excited and will want to visit. Your mother or mother-in-law may announce that she will be staying with you for a few weeks—even if an invite hasn't been extended!

Now is the time that you and your partner will have to decide whether your houseguests will actually be a help or a hindrance. You may have a great relationship with your in-laws but know they will only get in the way. Or, hopefully, they will contribute by cooking, cleaning, and helping with the baby. The same goes for your own parents. However you feel, be sure to have an agreement with your partner and express your wishes in advance.

If you welcome them with open arms, fantastic! But if you can't, be gentle when telling them that you don't want any out-of-town guests for at least a month after the baby is born. You and your husband should also agree that he communicates his wishes with his family and you with yours. That way, there isn't any conflict between both of you and your in-laws.

Ways to Express Wishes to Family and Friends

Here are some gentle ways to explain your wishes to family and friends about visiting:

- Be polite but firm. Some new parents, especially ones who have pushy families, can't get a simple "no" across, or if they do, those families are not listening. Explain lovingly but firmly that you are exhausted and you need some time to rest and recover before having visitors. Tell them you'll email photos or post pictures on Facebook or call them on the phone instead.

- Explain to family that you and your partner need time to bond with the baby, at least for the first few days at home. Say, "Baby and I are doing well, but we're getting to know each other, and I'm learning to breastfeed, so we will let you know when we are ready for visitors."

- If someone arrives unannounced and you're in the midst of having a meltdown, your lovely husband can intervene at the door with "I'm so sorry, Mom (or baby) just went down for a nap."

- If you're home alone, put a note on the door with a "DO NOT RING DOORBELL" sign so no one disturbs you or baby's naptime.

- Let friends and family know that you're making only outgoing phone calls for that first week or so and that your phone ringer will be off.

- Change your voicemail and email to let people know that you're off the grid for a little while. Say, "Thanks for your email (or call). We're getting used to being new parents, so be patient with us, as we may take some time getting back to you."

What to Say to Aunt Bessie (and Other Visitors You're Not Quite Ready For)

I think it's safe to say everyone has an aunt or uncle that is either (a) a loudmouth, (b) offensive, (c) bossy, or (d) attention seeking. For these "special" people, you may need a little more than common sense replies. They won't take "no" for an answer, and their visits always end up with someone getting offended or into an argument. So here are some things to say in these particular cases. (Note: little white lies are totally acceptable.)

- Tell your bossy relative that your doctor has recommended that you limit/not have visitors until a week or two afterward. Say that the doctor is concerned about the risk of infection after your difficult birth. Relatives will believe the doctor, right?! You can even have the doctor write a note if you can't bear the little taradiddle.

- The pediatrician is concerned about germs and is recommending that guests don't visit until after at least four weeks. Yes, you're upset too! But you shouldn't go against doctor's orders!

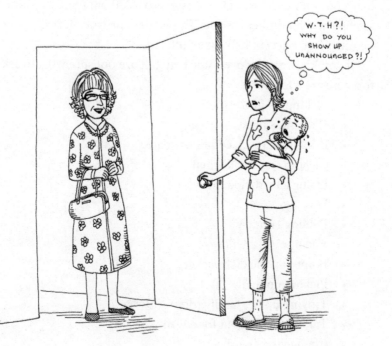

- Uncle Lucas shows up at your doorstep with the entire soccer team of kids. Dad can answer the door and tell the brood that mom has taken baby to the pediatrician's office for a checkup. Tell Uncle Lucas that it's probably best to call to make sure they're home first.

When You Are Ready

If your immediate family is coming to visit soon after birth, you may want to welcome them as long as they don't just visit but also offer help if you need it. I struggled those first few weeks after giving birth, and the only assistance I wanted was from my mom. I wasn't ready to have other family members and friends over just yet.

If a family member or friend asks if you need anything, say "YES!" Don't be shy about asking them to bring your favorite soup or meal. Some people are just itching to help when you have a baby, but they don't want to overstep, so ask them to tidy up your kitchen or start dinner for you. This is the time when it really does take a village—accept help when offered.

If you know you'd love some help but are not sure what to ask for, here are a few ideas:

- Picking up groceries
- Cooking a meal
- Bringing a meal, coffee, or snacks
- Cleaning up the kitchen
- Doing a load of laundry
- Dusting
- Folding laundry
- Vacuuming the floors
- Emptying the dishwasher
- Picking up mail
- Tidying up the family room
- Taking the dog out for a walk
- Change the bed sheets

If your visitor is not asking "What can I to help?" but you could really use a hand, this is the time to shamelessly ask. I find that some family and friends who may not have kids don't know *how* to help; they may not realize that a small task such as checking the mail or picking up some eggs and milk is a tremendous help to you. Put your pride aside and simply ask, "Could you do me a huge favor?"

This tip works well for friends who want to visit you and baby: ask, "Would you mind picking up a Starbucks for me on the way?" Bonus—your friends will bring a coffee for themselves too.

Short and Sweet

Once you are ready for other visitors, which may be after several weeks have passed, make sure family and friends realize they may have only minutes to hold your baby in between naps and feedings. Make it clear that the visit will be short. Give specific times; for example, "Baby will eat and nap around one o'clock in the afternoon, so if you arrive at three o'clock for a quick hour, that would work best."

Ask anyone who is ill to not step foot into your home until they are in the clear. Ask visitors to wash their hands before holding your baby—a newborn's immune system is not fully developed.

Don't be shy about reminding your guests that you are tired and need time to rest. It is totally acceptable to leave it to your partner to gently tell them it's time for them to go. Here are some things you could say to gently remind your guests they've overextended their stay:

- "I think I need to nurse the baby and rest for a while. I'm sorry to leave you now, but it was great seeing you. Thanks for coming by."
- "Gosh, I only slept a total of three hours last night; I'm exhausted. Please excuse me, but I have to go to my bedroom and take a nap."

- "The doctor said I have to limit visitors because of my surgery/recovery. I wish I could have you stay longer!"
- "I'd love to have you stay for lunch, but we're still getting used to all of this and haven't cooked a proper meal yet!"
- For those visitors who show up at your doorstep, gently tell them, "We love that you want to stop by, but it would be great to call first so the baby and I don't both sleep through your visit."

It would also be helpful if your partner is on the ball and able to help when it's time to cut the visit short. You could even come up with a code word, gesture, or simply a big yawn to let him know that it's time to say goodbye to your guests. New Dad could easily tell Mom, "Honey, you and the baby should go upstairs to rest for a bit." If that doesn't hint to guests that they've overstayed their welcome, Dad can say, "Well, it was so great seeing you! Hopefully next time you can stay a bit longer."

If any of those tips don't work, then give your lingering guest the boot! Stand up and say, "Let me walk you to the door. It's time I got some rest." You may need to guide your guest ever so gently by the elbow up and OUT. Just smile as you send them on their way.

Traditions

In some cultures, it may be tradition to have the entire family, including third and fourth cousins, drop by to welcome the baby. In this case, the entire village is in your house to celebrate baby's arrival. You've lost this battle, but look on the bright side: you have a million hands to help out!

In some cultures, relatives must visit out of respect for the family. I understand that this would make your parents happy and proud, but this isn't about them—it's about you, your husband, and the baby. The last thing I was in the mood for were distant relatives coming over and just *staring* at me and the baby simply because they knew visiting was the respectful thing to do. There will always be time several weeks later to meet distant relatives and friends of the family.

Many cultures around the world believe in a period of rest for the mother and the baby after the birthing process. In Japan, women remain in bed with the newborn for three weeks while visiting with people wanting to see the new baby. In Chinese culture, the mother is required to *zuo yuezi,* or stay in bed, for a month in order to recover from the fatigue. In this month, she is advised to stay at home and not go outdoors for fear of negative effects on her health.

The same tradition holds true for my mom's generation of Greeks. A Greek mother is often expected to stay at home with her newborn baby for forty days after the birth of a child. She isn't supposed to go out, even to the grocery store, and if she is lucky enough to have family support, she doesn't cook or clean or do any of her normal household duties. The only time that a new mother leaves the house is for a doctor's appointment. Once the forty days have passed, Mom and baby will attend church and receive a blessing known as *Sarantismos,* the forty-day blessing.

These traditions bring families and peoples together. They are often healing—when else can you stay in bed for a month? While respecting your culture, remember to speak up for yourself if your needs do not entirely match others' ideas. Whatever your family and cultural traditions are, embrace this time of bonding, recovery, and rest.

Mom to Mom

I asked some moms how quickly they allowed visitors. Here are their replies:

I wanted no visitors at the hospital until a few hours after babe was born (other than immediate family), and this was great for bonding with little one. As for home, I wanted visitors right away, but I was unable to due to postpartum preeclampsia. As soon as I was better, it was nice getting out and seeing people to share my little miracle, plus all the helping hands [were] great! —Lisa Cosentino

Only my family came to see me at the hospital. I didn't message any of my friends to let them know that I had the baby until after I was home. Once I was home, I think they came visiting on the second and third day. —Karen May

I gave birth in the hospital but had a midwife both times. The first time, everyone and their dog was in there shortly after the birth. The second time, I had only close family there but stayed in the hospital an extra night just to be alone with baby. —Heidi Hoile

I've always stuck to immediate family only in the hospital and by arrangement afterwards. Most people understand if you say, "Can you come Tuesday? Things are a bit crazy, and I'd like to be lucid when you first visit!" Mostly, it's important to assess how you feel and how you want to do it. Be selfish; if you want to show baby off, DO IT! If you don't, people worth their salt will understand. —Anjali Joshi

My parents were there with us when my son was born at eight o'clock in the morning; we had midwives, so we headed home by noon; my girlfriend and her husband brought us lunch and we had a picnic on my bed. Later, my siblings and parents all came for dinner (they brought it) because it was my husband's birthday. Everyone else called. I only told one person that it wouldn't work for her to visit because we weren't super close and it would have felt too much like entertaining. —Janelle Dayman

I had the people closest to me visit at the hospital the day after baby was born. She was born really late at night, so that gave me some time alone with my hubby and baby. The first week at home, I really didn't want anyone visiting. I wanted to find my new normal and recover a bit first.
—Kelley Scott Driediger

I had my daughter in the evening, and we had our parents and siblings come meet her the next morning. Everyone else met her once we were home from the hospital. Prior to her birth, we had warned our families that the time of day she was born would determine when we allowed visitors. We explained that we needed time for the three of us to bond as a family before we could have others. I also explained that I wanted some private time with my daughter for skin-to-skin and to establish breastfeeding before visitors came. Our experience was that we were ready for our families to visit within about twelve hours of her birth. —Liora Sobel

Hospital: just close family. I told everyone else that I was too tired for visitors. Home: just close family right away. I told everyone else we needed a couple of weeks, that things [were] too busy at the moment. —Nicole Kalbfleisch

With my first, we welcomed immediate family at the hospital and cousins and friends at the house the day we got home. With my second, we had just my parents at the hospital and visitors about a month later (with the exception of one girlfriend). I was so tired the second time around with a newborn and a toddler in the house! —Marlene Nemeth

Chapter Three

THIS DIDN'T COME WITH INSTRUCTIONS

Now you're home and thinking: *What next? Can I re-member everything I read in my pregnancy books? The nurses demonstrated some breastfeeding techniques, but I can't even remember how to help my baby latch on properly. With so many things to remember for my newborn baby, I wonder, am I doing the right thing? I feel like I don't have a clue!*

First, take a deep breath and know that you're not the only new parent feeling overwhelmed. It doesn't matter how many baby books you've read or videos you've watched; it's another ball game when you're experiencing something for yourself the first time. But there's a first time for everything, and you'll quickly get the hang of things, including changing a diaper, giving baby a bath, cutting those tiny little fingernails, and finding just how baby likes to be soothed.

Baby's-Now-Home Quick Checklist

- Newborns should eat eight to twelve times a day.
- Your baby may lose up to one-tenth of his birth weight during his first five days of life. But not to worry—he'll gain it back by day ten.
- Once babies have gained back their weight, falling asleep or turning away usually means they are full.
- Expect at least four wet diapers a day and one or more poopy diapers.
- If you breastfeed, poop will be mustard colored.
- If you formula-feed, poop will be yellow or tan.
- If you've had a C-section, take it easy. You must rest and limit your activity.
- The umbilical cord will dry up and fall off by about two weeks. Until then, keep it clean and fold down the diaper so the cord stays dry. You can give baby sponge baths until the cord falls off.
- If you breastfeed, you may feel hungrier, as your body is producing milk. Make sure to eat healthy meals and stay hydrated.
- When baby comes home, keep it noisy. There's no need to have a quiet house; in fact, it's better to maintain the same volume so that baby will get used to the noise level.

Changing Baby's Diaper

Who knew that baby's poop could fly across a room? And that it would have strange colors?! Newborn poop is mostly liquid with some mustard-seed texture mixed in it. Mustard-seed texture as in bright yellow with sesame seeds inside—or something like that. (Eww.) When it's your baby, though, of course you don't mind . . . unless you're changing diapers all the time. Did you know that sometimes you'll have to change your baby's diaper every hour?!

You may feel completely uncoordinated when you attempt to change baby's diaper the first few times. *How do I hold baby's legs up to wipe his bum? What do I do with the dirty diaper? There really should be some sort of automated machine for this task!*

Once you've cleaned and changed baby and put his clothes back on, you hear *Ppppprrrrrr*—a big wet poop. Again. Back to the diaper station! Luckily, though, newborn poop doesn't stink. That comes later when they start to eat more solid foods. Then you'll need a nose plug when you change your toddler's bum!

Make sure to have a crapload (pun intended) of diapers on hand. Whether you're buying disposable diapers or doing

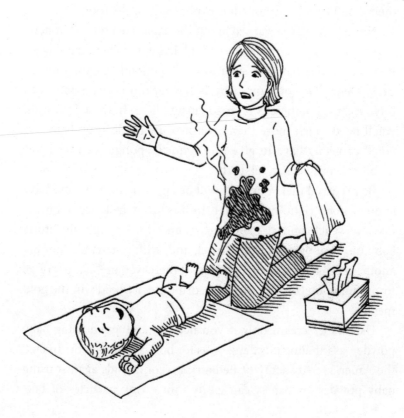

washable cloths, have them ready to go before baby arrives. Baby will go through them like Momma goes through a pot of coffee.

Some babies love being naked! They'll kick their legs and smile at you. Others don't like the process and will cry and squirm until the last snap is fastened. You can try hanging a mobile right above the change table to keep them occupied; my little one was entranced by his. He would stop any movement and lay there mesmerized, watching the mobile go 'round and 'round while I cleaned his cute little bum.

Tip: when you remove the diaper and put a fresh one on, be sure to *immediately* cover the baby's genitals, especially boys . . . otherwise, you may be sprayed! That sensation of cool air on your baby's penis will cause a fountain of pee. You'd be surprised by their aim. I swear, my boy hit the other side of the room!

Now, I was never warned about the *explosive* poops that newborns can create—I mean, like a bomb has gone off in their diaper. Poop can come out with such force, it can end up going up his back. Depending on how baby is laying, those disposables can leave a gap—oh, there is no road closure here. In these instances, you'll need much more than a warm wipe to clean up baby . . . you'll probably have to give him a quick sponge bath, or if his umbilical cord is off, a full bath.

Be prepared that your baby will be enjoying his bath and have another poop right in the water. In this lovely instance, I'd practice my synchronized hand movements by strategically lifting baby up, wrapping him in a towel, and, with one hand, running another bath to clean him up again. If there was an Olympic prize for cleaning up baby's poop in record time, I would win the gold medal.

Use diaper cream only if you need it, and avoid using baby powder, as inhaling it is dangerous for both you and baby. In fact, the American Academy of Pediatrics recommends against using baby powder, as babies can easily inhale tiny particles of talc, which are light enough to be carried in the air. When inhaled, talc can dry an infant's mucous membranes, affect the baby's breathing, and cause lung damage.

Changing diapers is an acquired skill. Before you know it, you'll be a pro!

How to Make a Baby Poop:

1. Change diaper
2. Dress baby in a fresh outfit
3. Wait one minute

Getting Baby Dressed

Dressing baby the first few times will feel like a gong show. Your baby will seem like an octopus with four arms and four legs! Babies aren't keen on being cold, and they don't like being pushed and pulled through clothing. Look for clothing that snaps or zips all the way down the front and both legs to make changes easier. Look for loose-fitting sleeves so your hand fits inside to pull baby's arm through. Avoid clothing with ribbons, strings, tight bands, and unbreathable materials.

I loved the button-up sleepers because I wouldn't have to pull anything over baby's head. There will be times when you or your spouse will screw it up and get the buttons all wrong, with extra buttons somehow not aligned right by baby's crotch! You'll then have to start all over again while trying to keep baby occupied. Here's where that mobile comes in handy. Also, sing and talk to your baby as you dress her. Baby loves the sound of your voice.

To easily get baby dressed, try laying him down. Next, lay the garment down beside baby, and then place baby on top of it. If you do have to pull a onesie over baby's head, stretch the garment neckline first and then pull it over while continuing to stretch it out so it doesn't catch on his sweet face. Place your hand into the sleeve from the outside, grasp your baby's hand, and pull it through. As you place legs inside sleepers, don't be surprised when those little knees and toes pop right back out before you have a chance to snap them in. This is when you wish you were the one with eight arms!

Baby's First Bath

For the first few weeks, you'll only need to sponge-bathe your sweet babe just a few times a week. After the umbilical cord stump dries up and falls off and the area heals, you can start giving your newborn a bath every few days. A baby bathtub will be helpful those first few months before baby can sit up in a bath chair. Have your bath supplies handy in a basket by the tub *before* you start; otherwise, you'll have to wrap baby in a towel mid-bath to find the soap. I like to lay baby's towel out so I can quickly place him on the towel and wrap him up for warmth. There's nothing worse than trying to hold a slippery, wet, screaming baby while unfolding the towel. Don't forget the camera! While either you or hubby holds the baby, the other will want to snap some photos of your little ducky swimming in the water.

Fill the tub with just a few inches of warm water. Before you put your baby in the bath water, test the water's temperature on the inside of your wrist to make sure it is not too hot. Using one arm to gently support your baby's back, head, and neck, gently place her in the baby bath.

With one hand always on baby, use the other to pour cupfuls of bath water over her regularly during the bath so she doesn't get too cold.

Using mild soap, gently cleanse around your baby's eyes with a cotton pad dampened with clean, warm water. Then wipe around your baby's mouth, nose, and whole face with a soft washcloth. Wipe the creases in her neck, and don't forget behind her ears!

Continue washing baby from top to bottom and the genital area from front to back. This is another time you'll wish you had four pairs of hands—they are slippery little suckers! Once bath time is done, quickly wrap baby in a towel and pat-dry her skin, including those cute little creases!

While bath time is meant to clean, it's also a special time for you to bond with your little monkey. It boosts the parenting bond. This is an ideal time to have Daddy participate. Watching your baby feel the water on him, kissing his chubby rolls, hearing him splash his little hands in the water, tickling his little toes—is there anything cuter? If you're breastfeeding exclusively, bath time could be baby-daddy time for one-on-one bonding.

Bathing also helps soothe fussy babies and is a fantastic way to start a bedtime routine. Starting sleepy time off with a warm bath and towel is sure to induce a restful sleep. (Heck, I'd love for someone to wash my hair and then tuck me into clean-smelling jammies. Can I also be read a bedtime story?) The nightly routine will help reinforce the message that it's almost time for sleep . . . because soon after, you'll want to be sleeping too.

Baby's Skin and Cradle Cap

Your baby's skin may not be as flawless as you expect or see in media images. Smooth and soft newborn skin? Well, that is just not usually the case. Some babies have baby acne: little bumps and pimples. Hey, wait; doesn't that come in the teenage years along with puberty and raging hormones?! Neonatal acne may be caused by exposure in the womb to maternal hormones. It can last for weeks or even months, but don't fret; no treatment is needed, as baby's skin will clear up over time.[1]

How can your baby have dandruff? What the heck is this flaky stuff? If your baby's scalp has flaky, dry skin that looks like dandruff or thick, oily, yellowish or brown scaling or crusting patches, it's probably cradle cap. Cradle cap is more like cradle *crap*! This flaky scalp can also spread behind the ears and neck. I had no idea that babies could have these issues. Cradle cap usually clears up on its own within a few months.[2] A mild shampoo can help loosen and remove the scales. First, wet the scalp and then gently scrub with a soft-bristle brush. You can also try removing the scales gently with a fine-tooth comb. Rinse baby's head well and gently towel-dry. If the cradle cap starts spreading to other body parts, see your doctor.

Umbilical Cord

The stump left after the umbilical cord is cut will look weird and, perhaps, gross to you. It will change from bluish white to black as it dries out and eventually falls off, usually within three weeks after birth. The process of the cord changing colors and then falling off can cause concern, but it's normal. If the navel area becomes red, or if a foul odor or discharge develops, see your doctor. If you're using disposable diapers, fold the top of the diaper down so it doesn't rub against the cord. Give baby only sponge baths until the stump falls off. Babies don't smell bad anyway—they are blessed with that wonderful newborn baby smell. (Don't you wish you could just bottle that?) Don't attempt to pull the stump off—it really will just fall off.

What perfume am I wearing? It's a mix of green bamboo tea and baby spit-up.

Spit-Up

Your clothes will be stained and full of spit-up for the first few months, so be prepared to live in your sweatpants, yoga pants, T-shirts, and sweatshirts. If you're smart and manage to have burping pads handy, you'll save your wardrobe, so no excuse to buy a new one. (Your partner will love that.)

The American Academy of Pediatrics' *Caring for Your Baby and Young Child* advises to burp your baby every three to five minutes during feedings. Also, hold your baby in an upright position right after feeding. Burp your baby after every two to three ounces from the bottle or when she changes breasts.[3] Don't be startled by the loud belches that will come out of such a tiny baby. How can a little cutie pie create such beer-belching sounds? Soon enough, your hubby will be doing burping contests with baby.

Getting a burp out of your little thing is probably the greatest satisfaction I've come across. It's truly one of life's most satisfying moments. —Brad Pitt

Swaddle

If I knew what the real world was like, I would have wanted to stay in my mother's womb too. Your baby will miss the comfort and warmth of your womb. Aww! Swaddling your baby in a blanket and holding him in your arms makes him feel protected. I remember my little one would be so startled by his own movements when I was changing his diaper. All of a sudden, he'd bust into a "Yo!" hip-hop pose, with his little hands up in the air and his fingers spread. "Put yo' hands up in the air, and wave 'em like you just don't care!"

Your Baby & Child by Penelope Leach suggests securely wrapping baby so that he will not wake even during the normal periods of light sleep.[4] Keep him face up to reduce the risk of SIDS. Your newborn's internal thermostat still doesn't work very well either, so you'll want to keep him dressed with one more layer than what you would wear—but not more. Baby does not need a sweat bath.

Baby Burrito

1. Lay a thin blanket in a diamond shape. Fold top corner down and place baby on top.
2. Pull one side of blanket across baby's chest and tuck under opposite arm.
3. Fold bottom of blanket over feet and tuck behind baby's shoulder.
4. Pull corner above baby's shoulder, fold down over shoulder, and tuck in blanket fold.
5. Pull remaining side of blanket across the baby's chest, continuing around baby, and secure under blanket.

Properly swaddled, your cozy and content baby may even fall asleep—yay!

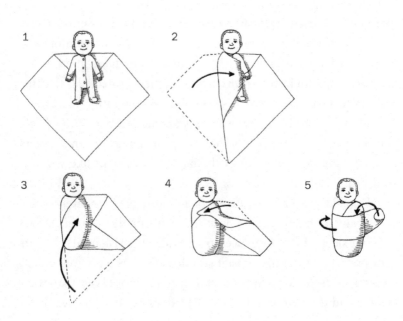

Reflexes

Newborns have several reflexes, which are involuntary movements or actions. While you may be wondering why your baby is twitching or shooting his arms out at odd times, these are actually signs that everything is working just fine. Many of these innate responses will disappear in a few months as your baby's body and brain develops.

The Moro reflex is often called a startle reflex because it usually occurs when a baby is startled by a loud sound or movement. Baby will throw out her legs and arms and then pull them back in. It's like baby is doing the Elaine dance from the TV show *Seinfeld*.

You will have endless fun testing out the walking (or stepping) reflex as you hold your baby up with his legs dangling on the floor or bed. Try it! He will place one foot in front of the other and start to walk in place. I remember laughing when my baby did this, asking him, "Where are you going?!" Be sure to support baby's head and body when trying this.

My favorite reflex is when you stroke the side of your baby's cheek with your fingers or breast and your baby automatically turns his head toward it. He'll open his mouth to follow, rooting in the direction of the stroking and beginning to make sucking movements. This is the most basic of survival instincts and helps the baby find the breast to latch onto or the bottle to begin feeding. It's the most adorable reflex to watch in action.

You may feel a little off balance as you settle into life as a mom. From reflexes to diapering and bathing baby, everything is new. Just as learning to ride a bicycle takes some practice, so does caring for an infant. Once you feel comfortable enough to take the training wheels off, you'll feel confident to ride down the hill!

Mom to Mom

Diapering Disasters

When my son was five weeks old, we moved into a new house with a separate apartment (which was vacant). My husband had just finished staying up all night painting the house while my son and I slept in the vacant apartment. It was five o'clock a.m. when my husband finally finished painting and lay down to sleep. Not two minutes after, I heard gas noises from my little guy's diaper. After waiting a minute and thinking he was finished, I took him to the changing table for a fresh diaper. I opened the diaper, and, to my surprise, it was empty. Then I heard the noises again and quickly tried to do up that diaper. But I was too late. Poo flew across the room and sprayed all over my husband's back. I stood there frozen, watching the poo everywhere, and then my husband and I started laughing instantly. No one tells you about the flying poop accidents when you're a new parent. —Kristen Stevens

My husband and I are hockey fans, he a Bruins fan and I a Leafs fan. When my mom was staying with me for the first few weeks to help out, I was changing my son's diaper and had his legs up in the air. Suddenly, out comes the flying poop. I never squealed so loud! While still trying to hold him, I attempted to dodge the stream, but it was inevitable: projectile all over me and my Leafs blanket! My mom and I laughed so loud! My hubby likes to tease me, saying our son likes his dad's team better and he proved that my team stinks. —Tasha Harps

What Moms Found to Be Most Challenging with Their Newborn:

The hardest for me was always feeling like she wasn't eating enough . . . I always second-guessed myself. —Melissa Gropp Pourgoutzidis

Nail clipping! Even after four newborns, I am still not used to or comfortable with clipping their nails. It's a job for steady-handed Daddy in our house. —Jennifer Walker

I was terrified to drive in the car with her—I was a single mom at forty-two with an incredible sales career, but the moment I had to drive with Ella in the car, the anxiety was overwhelming. —Amy Riddell-Catney

The first bath was more awkward and nerve racking than hard. My baby was just so tiny and screaming because he was cold and afraid. It makes you feel like you're doing something wrong.—Emily Strawbridge

Chapter Four

BREASTFEEDING DOES *NOT* COME NATURALLY

You see images of blissfully nursing new mothers breastfeeding their cherub-like rosy-cheeked babes and think *Breastfeeding looks so natural.* You would think breastfeeding was an innate skill. What could come as naturally to a new mama and baby than to give and take nourishment from a swollen breast?

But for many, breastfeeding is more difficult than it looks—as I quickly discovered. The reality is, for most women (and new babies), breastfeeding takes a lot of patience and hard work.

My eldest had trouble latching, while I suffered multiple bouts of mastitis with my youngest. This wasn't the vision I'd had of breastfeeding my newborn. I thought breastfeeding would be effortless. Natural. Beautiful. Instead, it was a real challenge.

What They Didn't Tell You

- Your nipples will crack and bleed as you learn how to position properly to get a better latch.
- Your breasts will feel beaten and swollen as they engorge with milk and then empty out after feedings.
- Squeezing your breasts to release some of the buildup will feel as good as peeing after keeping a full bladder for an abdominal ultrasound.

The good news is, with a little guidance and a lot of practice, breastfeeding does get easier. It will likely become a source of nourishment and comfort for your baby, just as you dreamt it would be.

Nursing moms who breastfeed like pros will tell you it is the best way to make sure your baby gets the nutrition they need and antibodies to protect them. They'll tell how it helps you lose weight after giving birth. And they will speak of how beautifully they bond with their baby as she suckles.

> *Breastfeeding is nature's health plan. —Author unknown*

Still, there are difficult parts that nobody warned me about. Nobody told me about the cracking, sore nipples or wrestling with a breast pump or squirming to find a comfortable position. But when you're determined to breastfeed your baby, you'll do whatever it takes—for some, the difficulties are a small price to pay for the benefits. Those moms who didn't warn you forgot the pain, because the joy outweighed every challenge they experienced.

Breastfeeding brings so many emotions to the surface. As mothers, we want to provide the best nourishment for our babies. Then when it doesn't come naturally, we wonder: *Why does something that is supposed to be wonderful and natural feel so difficult?*

Nursing Early

Breastfeeding was, without question, something I was determined to do. It wasn't even a decision I made—it was an innate knowing. I knew that it would take time and practice, and I was willing to do whatever it took to make it work. So I was furious when my son's first taste of milk was not my own.

Since he was taken away and put on IV antibiotics, rather than bring him to me and put him to my breast, the doctors decided to feed him milk from a dropper. Why would they do that? The nursery staff told me they figured I needed the rest and he needed to eat. But I was still furious about not having the opportunity to decide for myself. After all, I was the baby's mother! Be sure to communicate your feeding plans to your hospital so you can make your own choices.

Studies show that a breastfeeding newborn who has early contact with their mother learns to latch on more efficiently than a baby who is separated from their mother in the hour or two following birth.[5]

As much as you can in the first few days, lay your baby on your chest only in his diaper. The skin to skin will cue him to breastfeed more often. A baby who nurses frequently in the first few days (more than eight times in twenty-four hours) will help your milk supply. Plus, baby won't lose too much weight and is less likely to develop jaundice. The more you breastfeed, the faster your milk will come in, so frequent feeds in the first days will help milk production.

The International Breastfeeding Centre (IBC) recommends skin-to-skin contact immediately after birth for at least an hour and as often as possible throughout baby's first weeks. According to IBC, skin-to-skin contact has the following positive effects:

- Baby is more likely to latch on and latch on well.
- Baby maintains his normal body temperature better even than an incubator.

- Baby maintains his heart rate, respiratory rate, blood pressure, and blood sugar.
- Baby is less likely to cry.
- Baby is more likely to breastfeed exclusively and breastfeed longer.
- Baby will indicate to his mother when he is ready to feed.[6]

At the time, I was devastated that I wasn't given this opportunity to bond with my baby. When I finally had the chance to hold my baby and feed him, he took to my breast right away—or so I thought.

The first few days, your breasts excrete colostrum, which is not quite milk yet but full of nutrients for baby. Your breasts actually begin producing colostrum during pregnancy. It's thick, sticky, yellow/orange in color, and high in carbohydrates, protein, and antibodies to help keep your baby healthy. It's easy for baby to digest and low in volume but high in concentrated nutrition for your newborn. Babies need only a few milliliters per feed at this early stage.

It feels like the baby is sucking and nothing is coming out, but it is! This is when those early frequent feedings come in. Remember to feed at least eight to twelve times each day. This allows your baby to get all the benefits of the colostrum and also stimulates production of a plentiful supply of mature milk.

Latching

Before baby can enjoy her milk, she must get a proper latch on your breast. Getting this right from the start is essential. I never thought there was an art to getting baby to latch. Seriously, no one told me this. I thought baby would simply start to suckle at mom's breast, eat, and be merry. But I soon realized getting baby to latch properly is a science. Like an alligator, my baby would open his mouth wide and chomp down. Ouch!

It's normal for your nipples to feel a bit tender the first few days as they accustom to breastfeeding and the skin toughens. But breastfeeding shouldn't hurt. I had to see a lactation nurse because my nipples were badly cracked: a sign of an improper latch.

If your baby tends to suck on the tip of your nipple without getting much of your areola, he is latched on incorrectly. You'll need to fix this right away. Baby's little mouth should be as open as possible so the whole areola can fit in baby's mouth with the nipple at the roof of his mouth. If he's sucking only on the nipple, you will get cracked and bleeding nipples. Let me tell you: it's quite painful! On top of nursing, you'll have to also treat your breasts for risk of infection.

If you have a chance at the hospital to see a lactation consultant, I highly recommend it. Even if you think *Oh, I got this* or *I have had enough exposure to perfect strangers*, have a specialist take a look to ensure that baby is nursing effectively. An improper latch can be painful for you and ineffective for baby.

When the Milk Comes

It's tough to know what to expect when you have not yet experienced your milk *come in*. Will it end up feeling like a faucet you turn on; suddenly milk starts gushing everywhere? I mean, how do you know?

Your breasts will begin producing mature milk around the third or fourth day after birth. The milk will increase in volume and will appear thinner and whiter (opaquer) in color compared to the earlier thick, yellow colostrum.

When the milk does finally arrive, YOU JUST KNOW. Your breasts become rock hard and they start to ache until baby nurses. I remember coaxing my baby, "That's it—suck it dry! Get it all out!"

Those first few days, babies are very sleepy eaters. They will love to nuzzle into mom's breasts and nod off. It's important to keep baby awake while nursing. You'll know if she is by the loud swallowing sound. Rub baby's feet, back, or head to keep her nursing.

It can feel exhausting to nurse so frequently, but it will be worth it. The more work you put into breastfeeding now, the better milk supply later. Part of that breastfeeding work involves eating healthy . . . and often. Those early days of breastfeeding will leave you ragged and hungry. My mom, God bless her soul, brought me food. Lots of fresh, home-cooked food, like her delicious Greek chicken soup. I would eat bowls of it, like I had never eaten before. Maybe it was a Greek tradition to eat this magical chicken soup after giving birth, because I remember Mom insisting, "Eat this; it'll help with your milk." And the milk did come . . . boy, did it ever!

Chicken Soup Avgolemono (Egg Lemon Soup)

Ingredients:

　　3–4 chicken breasts with bone
　　2–3 carrots (each cut into 2–3 pieces)
　　2 celery stalks (cut in half)
　　2–3 onions (leave whole if small, or cut in half)
　　1 teaspoon salt
　　Peppercorns (about 6 or so)
　　1 cup rice
　　1–2 eggs
　　1 lemon, juice squeezed

Directions:

1. Boil chicken breast in a five-quart pot until cooked. Spoon away the foam. In the same pot, add carrots, celery, onions, salt, and peppercorns. Cook until vegetables are tender. Remove chicken and vegetables and put aside, leaving broth behind.

2. Add more water to the pot if needed to fill pot about halfway and cook until boiling. Add rice. Continue on a low boil, uncovered, for about 20 minutes. Once rice is cooked, turn off the heat.

3. In a bowl, beat egg whites until foamy, into a meringue. Then beat in the yolks. Add lemon juice and beat. Then add some broth and beat again.

4. Cut pieces of chicken into cubes or small pieces. Cut vegetables as well—if you desire, use a hand blender to chop, then add to the pot with the rice. Then pour egg/lemon mixture into pot with rice. Turn heat on for a few minutes until soup begins to boil. Serve! Eat up!

5. This soup freezes well, so if you have leftovers, divide up into single servings and freeze. Thaw in refrigerator for a quick meal.

How Often Will Baby Nurse?

Before your milk supply is established, breastfeeding should be *on demand* (when your baby is hungry), which is generally every one-and-a-half to three hours. Your newborn should be nursing eight to twelve times per day for about the first month. By one to two months of age, a breastfed baby will probably nurse eight to nine times a day.[7]

As newborns get older, they'll nurse less often and may develop a more reliable schedule. Some babies may nurse every ninety minutes, while others may go two or three hours between feedings. Newborns should not go more than about four hours without feeding, even during the night.

Because my baby was still learning to nurse—and so was I—feedings took a long time. My son would be on the breast for a good forty minutes, it seemed. By the time my hungry boy finished sucking and being burped and diaper-changed, he was fast asleep again. Then, before I knew it, he was up and ready for another feeding.

I obviously wasn't a pro yet, so getting up to feed at night was a challenge! Teaching my son to latch properly—sitting up with a nursing pillow, all the while half asleep—was no piece of cake. Nursing at night seemed like a long process.

It may feel as though you're feeding your little one more often than a fellow new mom whose baby is formula-fed. Breast milk digests easier than formula, which means it moves through your baby's digestive system faster. So your baby will be hungry more often, and, lucky you, there will be more diapers to change.

In the beginning, you may feel like you're nursing around the clock. When you measure the length of time in between feedings, count from the time when your baby begins to nurse (rather than when he or she ends) to the time when your baby starts nursing again. So if your first feeding started at eight o'clock in the morning and the next feeding was at around ten o'clock, that would count as every two hours.

Signs That Baby Is Hungry

Baby will:
- move head from side to side
- open mouth
- stick out tongue
- place hands and fists to mouth
- pucker lips as if to suck
- nuzzle against mother's breasts
- show the rooting reflex

Engorgement

Engorgement is when your breasts flood with milk and blood flows to your breasts, making the tissues swell. Your breasts will become engorged with milk and feel hot and sometimes painful. While it may be uncomfortable, this is perfectly normal. Your body is producing milk, and once your baby feeds regularly, the discomfort will pass.

The feeling as baby starts relieving some of that engorgement is like a dark sky opening and sunlight streaming through. It feels like a balloon that's about to burst; suddenly some air is released and it doesn't pop after all.

If breasts are engorged, not only is it painful, but also baby will have a hard time latching on to nurse. Especially when your milk first comes in, as well as any other time you produce more milk than baby can eat, use these tips to relieve symptoms:

- Soften your breasts before feedings by gently massaging them or by expressing a little milk first so that baby can get a better latch.
- Apply a warm compress for a couple of minutes before you breastfeed.
- Use cold compresses after feedings to help reduce swelling. You can use a frozen wet towel, a cold pack, or a bag of frozen vegetables.
- Breastfeed more often, or use a breast pump to soften severely engorged breasts.
- Gently massage and compress the breast when the baby pauses between sucks, which may help drain the breast completely.
- Ask your health care professional about medications such as ibuprofen to reduce pain and inflammation.

Wiki Fact

When the swelling goes down, the milk can flow more easily, relieving the engorgement. Reducing this inflammation makes mom much more comfortable. If you're engorged, simply place cabbage leaves (either chilled or at room temperature) on the skin of your breasts (stick them right in your bra).

Let-Down

The let-down reflex usually happens after your baby has been sucking the breast for about two minutes. Some moms can let down their milk right away, meaning the milk will begin to freely flow. When the let-down occurs, you'll hear the baby's swallowing change to big gulps to keep up with the flow of milk.

Sometimes your baby roots for your nipple, gets ahold, and starts to suck—but then lets go! Your nipple begins to spray sweet, warm milk everywhere. The best is when baby looks startled as the milk starts gushing all over his face!

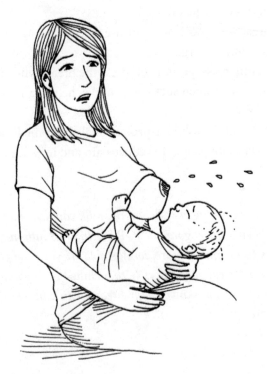

Milk Supply

Now where's that cowbell?

You will feel like a milk machine, for real. When your breasts fill up with milk and they begin to ache, a little squeeze—and suddenly it's Niagara Falls. The milk just keeps flowing—where the heck does it come from?! According to La Leche League, a full milk supply after two weeks is about thirty ounces every twenty-four hours.[8] That's about 1.6 gallons of milk per week!

It's amazing what your body can do, especially when your baby seems to require more milk. Your body will know to produce more nourishment for your baby. The more you produce, the more you need to keep eating, too. (Go make some chicken soup!)

I know many new mothers who worry they aren't producing enough milk. In most cases, yes, your baby is getting enough. You'll know baby is getting enough by the amount of wet diapers and steady weight gain. Counting your baby's diapers can be a helpful indicator as to whether or not he is getting enough of your milk. La Leche League says babies from one to six weeks old will have five to six wet diapers per day. Most babies will also have loose, bright yellow stools anywhere from three to five times a day. Some babies will have less frequent but larger stools.[9] If baby is losing weight or not having enough wet diapers, talk to your doctor.

Unfortunately, some moms encounter family members who feel they have a right to feed your baby. You may receive unsolicited advice from relatives: "You should give him formula from a bottle so you know how much he's eating." "How can I be a proper grandma if you don't let me give my grandbaby a bottle?" Our parents' generation was pushed to formula-feed. In the 1940s and 1950s, formula became a popular and safe substitute for breast milk, and breastfeeding experienced a steady decline. But in the 1970s, a movement began to promote breastfeeding, and it became popular once again.[10]

So, while Grandma may not agree with your choice to solely breastfeed, don't feel pressured to change. If you're successful in pumping your milk, you can save a bottle for Grandma or Auntie for some of their own bonding time. If you don't want to pump or offer a bottle, let Grandma know you'd love for her to burp baby and help dress or snuggle baby after a diaper change.

How Long Does It Take to Nurse?

How long babies nurse depends on several factors, including if your milk supply has come in completely, if your let-down reflex is immediate, and if your milk flow is slow or fast, as well as if your baby is latching properly and if your baby is sleepy.

As Mom becomes more confident with breastfeeding and baby becomes a professional, feedings will take less time. As you both become more efficient, feedings may take about five to ten minutes on each side, whereas newborns may feed for up to twenty minutes on each breast.

Alternating Breasts

It's important to alternate breasts when nursing to help keep your milk supply consistent and prevent painful engorgement. Some experts recommend switching breasts in the middle of each feeding and alternating which breast you offer first each time.

You may not remember on which breast your baby last nursed, so you can attach a small ribbon or safety pin to your bra strap to help or write it in a journal. You will be able to tell because one will feel more engorged than the other when it's time for the next feeding.

Positions

The breast pillow will be your best friend the first few weeks. Have a comfortable seating area and side table nearby set up for nursing since you'll be spending so much time there. You'll get to know what positions for feeding are most comfortable. My favorite position was the traditional one, but I also enjoyed the football position where baby's body would cradle my side rather than my chest.

Have a book, glass of water, breast cream, nursing pads, remote control for the TV, and your cell phone nearby. Otherwise, you'll be trying to reach for the remote with your feet!

Get Your Partner Involved

Even if you're breastfeeding, your partner can still help! If you're having trouble latching, hubby can help guide baby to latch properly. He can also prop you up with pillows, get you a glass of water, and then burp baby once fed. If you pump milk after nursing, you will be able to share a feeding with your husband—maybe even one of those middle-of-the-night feedings!

Don't Forget the Nursing Pads

Now that you and baby have the basics down and your milk supply is established, you will want to tuck nursing pads into your bra. There are times when your milk will let down when your baby is nowhere nearby. You can buy disposable or washable pads that absorb excess milk or catch a let-down when you are not prepared. You'll also find that when your milk lets down, both breasts will begin to flow milk. This creates a leaky side—unless you have twins!

Reusable breast pads are made with soft, washable material and feel nicer on your skin—especially if you have sore nipples. But the milk can go through quickly if you tend to leak a lot.

Disposable pads might be more absorbent. You may wish to try both types of nursing pads and see which you prefer.

One afternoon, we decided to have a nice family outing. I managed to throw on some makeup and nice clothes. I stumbled in my heels, trying to balance, and off we headed for some shopping. After an hour or so, we sat down for a cup of coffee. That's when I noticed. I looked down at my blouse and realized . . . I had two wet spots on my breasts. My breasts had leaked through the bra and onto my shirt! I had forgotten my pads. How embarrassing to not realize that I was walking around a busy shopping mall with two round stains on my shirt.

To Cover or Not to Cover?

I think this is a woman's choice. I know; there are many women out there who say breastfeeding in public can be normalized by *not* covering up. If you are comfortable with nursing in public, you'll be able to freely go out and enjoy. Breastfeeding in public shouldn't make anyone uncomfortable.

For some moms, it's not easy to go out and whip out a breast. If you're like me, you want to have a comfortable chair and nurse with ease, without onlookers. I was shy about my own body and nervous about my son's latch. My baby would tend to let go of my nipple often, so I preferred to have a nursing cover for use in public places for my own reasons. That was *my* choice. Because my baby wasn't an expert at latching, I often had to help him position his mouth properly. It would be a little awkward for me to be caught squeezing my breast and nipple, shoving it into the roof of a tiny baby's mouth! Plus, I'd often spray breast milk all over his face and, if someone was nearby, in their face too!

Do what you are most comfortable with, and don't feel pressured either way. If you do want to cover, there are darling cover-ups that you can slip around your neck so they don't blow off if you're at the park or they get pulled off by a wiggly baby. Just search online for cover-ups for nursing. They even make stylish nursing infinity scarves. We've come a long way, girls!

Bottle or Pacifier

If you plan to exclusively breastfeed, it's recommended to wait until breastfeeding is established before introducing a bottle or pacifier. Sucking on a bottle or a pacifier requires a different set of skills than breastfeeding. Experts suggest not introducing a bottle or pacifier to avoid nipple confusion until baby is three to four weeks old.

Once you've settled into a breastfeeding routine, keep in mind that sucking on a pacifier at naptime or bedtime might reduce the risk of SIDS.[11]

The caveat with this recommendation from the American Academy of Pediatrics is that some babies NEED to suck all the time, as it is a natural reflex for a newborn.[12] How can you satisfy their need to suck if you can't give baby a binky? Your breasts become the human pacifier! Also, if you have to wait several weeks before introducing a soother, then baby may not want it. Pay close attention to that tiny window of opportunity, or you will miss it completely.

That Time I Tried to Use a Hand Pump

I waited to introduce a bottle; as I experienced breastfeeding challenges, I went with the advice to avoid all artificial nipples for the first three to six weeks.

When my oldest son, the Boss, was about two months old, I tried pumping because I wanted to actually get out of the house without the baby. I didn't go out without the baby the first six weeks of his life—honest! But I knew there would come a time when I would need to spend longer periods of time without him right by my side. I was hopeful that pumping would be as easy as it looked. I figured I'd try a manual hand pump and see how it went. If baby took to the bottled breast milk, I'd consider moving up to an electric pump.

One morning, I opened the box and decided to put this thing together. You're supposed to attach this thingamajig to your breast and the milk goes into the bottle. Sounds easy enough, right? Well, I think I laughed the entire time I first used a handheld pump. "What are all of these parts?" I'm not even sure how I managed to put the thing together. If you're going to try pumping, do it solely for the scientific experimentation. It was interesting to watch how the nipple contorted into this device, how the milk would begin to release though the holes, and then to witness the let-down and how the milk would quickly stream out. Now I really felt like a cow!

I was victorious! I managed to pump a few ounces of milk. Then I went onto the next breast, which was aching for relief. When I removed the pump from my breast, I felt like my nipples had been stretched from here to Wyoming! Now that the milk was out of the breast and into the bottle, I handed it over to hubby to feed the Boss.

He gently waved the bottle in front of baby's face. He nudged the nipple against baby's lips, coaxing him to open his tiny mouth. After a little prodding, the Boss took the nipple in, but he appeared confused. *What is this? This isn't the texture of nipple I'm used to . . . I don't smell Mommy. Why is Daddy feeding me?*

After a few moments, POP! Baby spit the nipple out. Well, wouldn't you know, he wouldn't take the bottle! Nope, the bottle's nipple didn't feel like Mommy's, so although there was breast milk in the bottle, the bottle itself was not the right vehicle to deliver the goods.

I tried different nipples, ones that were supposed to "feel like real nipples." Well, bottle nipples don't look like Mommy's, and the material surrounding it feels like plastic. Every time my husband or I tried, he refused. *It's not as soft and warm as Mommy's boobies—you think I'm stupid?* Who was I trying to fool? This baby was smart. He wasn't going to be tricked into something he wasn't used to. (Don't blame you, kiddo. I'd be looking for Mom's boobies too.) For the next nine months, I was never much farther than a ten-minute drive from my baby.

I tried to pump my milk several times, but with a handheld, it took way too long. I don't know why I never thought of renting a pump, but I really didn't have to. I was home for a year; I didn't see the need to rent one if I was around. With the lack of success getting the Boss to even take the pumped milk, it seemed silly to spend money on one anyway.

Looking back, I had a tiny window of opportunity to introduce the bottle so that I could pump and allow others to feed baby. But I missed it! Introducing a bottle after establishing breastfeeding but before six weeks is the ideal time.[13] After that, baby may refuse to take a bottle from you if he can smell your breast milk. In this case, have someone else feed baby while you're not in the room. Also, give it a few tries until baby takes the bottle; be consistent and persistent. Baby will soon realize some of his feedings will have to be by the bottle.

> *It is only in the act of nursing that woman realizes her motherhood in visible and tangible fashion; it is a joy of every moment. —Honoré de Balzac*

While breastfeeding does not come naturally to some women, it's a skill that takes patience and practice. If you're determined to breastfeed but you're finding it challenging, keep trying; you may need some extra time and guidance to get it down to a fine art. The benefits to both you and baby are so worth persevering.

Mom to Mom

Breastfeeding most certainly did not come naturally to me. It took a visit from a La Leche teacher and three visits to the nursing clinic to finally figure it out. I had overactive let-down and would drown my son every time. I was taught to feed him lying down so it would fight gravity and come out slower until my milk regulated to his needs and he grew into my let-down. Three months of breastfeeding lying down! Finally felt comfortable enough to leave the house after that. Still, it was worth it for me. —Vickie Cuff

I really wanted to breastfeed my baby, but I felt a lot of pressure from some of my family to bottle-feed because I wasn't being fair to my husband or them. My husband was so supportive though. Even when I was in pain and wanted to give up after a C-section, he called a lactation consultant, and they got me on track. I successfully breastfed for thirteen months. —Lisa Cosentino

I have two girls, and I breastfed the first for a year and the second for two years. In the beginning, I never had trouble with the latch or anything. The difficult part was the responsibility of it. In the first months, it often felt like everything was on me, because I had the goods. Once they were older, and we had our rhythm, it was wonderful. I encourage people to stick with it. —Heidi Hoile

Right from the beginning, I knew I wanted to breastfeed. It was a healthier choice and also a big money saver. Because of my C-section, I was in the hospital for a few days. My milk hadn't come in, so the nurses suggested giving her some formula after I nursed. I really was against formula, but in the end, it was best for my daughter. Once my milk came in, we stopped with the formula, as she was finally back at her birth weight and steadily gaining more. I am happy I stuck it out. —Alicia Denne

I had no issues with breastfeeding; my little one weaned himself just after his first birthday. My only issue was too much milk, so I had to pump. The doctor said I could have fed ten kids, and, no, I am not well endowed. Our bond is amazingly strong, which I attribute to breastfeeding, and he is very cuddly still with his Mommy. —Pamela Bray-Crawford

I wouldn't have made it without the Jack Newman cream; once I got that, I was good to go. I've been lucky to have an excellent milk supply and a baby that latched quickly and easily. He is an enthusiastic eater—he has given me blood blisters and taken a chunk out of my nipple—but all in all, it's good. I pump so my husband and my mom can feed him too. This way I can have a break every now and then. I strongly believe I am fortunate to be able to breastfeed, but I genuinely believe as long as your child is loved, it doesn't matter at all how they are fed. As long as you both make it through the day, it's all good. —Lauren Tobin

Chapter Five

BREASTFEEDING BENEFITS AND TIPS ON FEEDING MOM, TOO!

Many medical authorities, including the American Academy of Pediatrics (AAP) and the American College of Obstetricians and Gynecologists, strongly recommend breastfeeding for the first six months of baby's life. There is simply no substitute for breast milk when it comes to protecting the health of your baby. Breast milk contains the exact amount of fat, sugar, water, and protein that your baby needs. Breast milk also contains antibodies, growth factors, essential fatty acids, and hormones that protect your baby from illness and help him develop at just the right pace. Breastfed babies have a reduced risk of many childhood diseases, including asthma, ear infections, intestinal infections, and allergies.

Among the known health benefits are: nutritionally balanced meals, some protection against common childhood infections, and better survival during the first year of life, including a lower risk of Sudden Infant Death Syndrome.[14] Studies also suggest that breastfeeding may reduce the risk for certain allergic diseases, asthma, obesity, and type 2 diabetes and may also may help improve an infant's cognitive development.[15]

Benefits for Mom

The benefits for baby are enough reason to breastfeed, but did you know there are also benefits for mom? Breastfeeding burns extra calories, so it can help you lose pregnancy weight faster. It releases the hormone oxytocin, which helps your uterus return to its pre-pregnancy size and may reduce uterine bleeding after birth. Breastfeeding also lowers your risk of breast and ovarian cancer.[16]

There are benefits beyond mom's health as well. Since you don't have to buy and measure formula, sterilize nipples, or warm bottles, it saves you time and money. It also gives you regular time to relax quietly with your newborn as you bond. I found it so convenient to just pop out my breast and feed on demand.

Formula-fed babies need about one to one and one-half cans of formula per week, with a can of powdered formula costing twenty to thirty dollars. If your baby requires special formula due to allergies or other special nutritional needs, formula feeding can cost around $250 per month. So your family could spend anywhere from $960 to $3,000 on formula in baby's first year! Instead of spending money on formula, you could use that money toward a college fund or a much-needed vacation.

Nutrition for Mom

The American Pregnancy Association says, "the higher the nutritional quality of the mom's diet, the higher the nutritional quality of the milk."[17] If you are breastfeeding, it's important to eat a healthy diet with foods rich in nutrients, drink plenty of water, and rest as much as possible.

Your nursing body is remarkably efficient at producing milk, so you shouldn't need to take in too many extra calories while breastfeeding. The American Academy of Pediatrics says breastfeeding moms have "an increased daily energy need of 450 to 500 calories a day that can be met by a modest increase in a normally balanced varied diet."[18] Think of this amount as about the equivalent of an extra snack or small meal a day. The best bet is to follow your hunger as a guide to how much food you'll need to eat per day.

Studies have shown that most healthy breastfeeding women maintain an abundant milk supply while taking in anywhere from 1,800 to 2,500 or more calories per day. Although you're eating more calories per day, you're also burning calories by breastfeeding. So it is quite common to lose weight while you're nursing. However, it isn't a great idea to go on a strict diet when you are breastfeeding. Instead, choose to eat healthy and exercise, and you won't have to count calories.

Breastfeeding usually gives you a big appetite. So if you don't feel like eating, it could be a sign that you need extra emotional support. Sometimes, women who have postpartum depression lose their appetite. If you're finding it a struggle to eat, see your doctor and talk about how you're feeling.

Remember, there's no need to go on a special diet while you're breastfeeding. Simply focus on making healthy choices—and you and your baby will reap the rewards.

Meal Ideas

Here are some healthy meal ideas for breakfast, lunch, dinner, and snacks:

Breakfast

- Whole-grain cereal with skim milk or low-fat milk and a piece of fruit
- Hard-boiled eggs with avocado on whole-grain toast and a piece of fruit
- Two eggs with two slices of turkey bacon
- Greek yogurt with honey and walnuts
- Steel-cut oats with banana slices and berries
- Low-fat granola and fruit

Lunch/Dinner

- Wrap with grilled chicken breast and vegetables
- Mixed green salad with boiled eggs, avocado, walnuts, and feta cheese
- Pasta with tomato sauce and mushrooms
- Grilled or broiled fish with broccoli and sweet potato mash
- Chicken breast with brown rice and vegetables
- Stir-fry with shrimp or chicken and steamed rice
- Quinoa salad with vegetables, pear, and feta cheese
- Steak with steamed vegetables and a baked potato
- Pork tenderloin skewers with Greek tzatziki and tomato salad

Snacks

- Homemade trail mix with nuts, dried fruit, and dark chocolate chips
- Cheddar cheese and an apple
- Apple slices with peanut butter
- Baby spinach and melted cheese in a whole-wheat wrap

- Smoothie with low-fat yogurt or milk and fresh or frozen fruit
- Hummus and fresh vegetables
- Pretzels with organic peanut butter
- Protein shake
- Almonds and dried figs

Vitamin Supplements and Herbal Remedies

It is a good idea to continue taking prenatal vitamins while you are breastfeeding. According to *Health Canada*, your nutrient needs do shift slightly from pregnancy to breastfeeding. For example, you need less iron during breastfeeding but more zinc.[19] Some doctors recommend a multivitamin with high doses of vitamin D if mom isn't getting enough. The Vitamin D Council says if nursing moms take a supplement with less than 5,000 IU of vitamin D each day, baby will need a vitamin D supplement.[20] While many women opt for their normal multi- or prenatal vitamin, there are postnatal vitamin supplements available specifically for breastfeeding women.

The American Academy of Pediatrics warns that you should use the same caution with herbal remedies as you do during pregnancy with over-the-counter or prescription drugs while breastfeeding.[21] Use them only with the advice of a health care professional.

Food Tips

A healthy, well-fed mom produces better milk. Choosing healthy foods throughout the day will help you feel more energetic. What new mom couldn't use an energy boost? Remember that when you aren't getting the needed nutrients from your diet, your body will provide them from your own stores. If you're not eating well, you will be feeling even more exhausted. Make sure you get all the nutrients you and your baby need.

Your breast milk is loaded with calcium to help your baby's bones develop, so it's important for you to eat enough calcium to meet your own needs. Dairy products are one of the best sources of calcium, protein, and vitamins B and D. Try including at least three cups of dairy each day in your diet.

A lack of iron can drain your energy levels, making it hard for you to keep up with the demands of a newborn baby. Nursing moms need to eat extra protein and vitamin B-12; choose iron-rich foods like red meat, dark leafy greens, iron-fortified cereals, cheese, and eggs.

Make sure you're consuming enough vitamins and nutrients by enjoying a veggie or fruit or both with each meal or snack. See some ideas above.

The American Heart Association says eating fish offers heart-healthy omega-3 fatty acids, but stay away from those that are high in mercury, including shark, swordfish, marlin, king mackerel, and tilefish.[22] Salmon, like other fatty fish, is loaded with a type of fat called DHA that is crucial to the development of your baby's brain and nervous system, according to the Harvard T. H. Chan School of Public Health.[23] Limit canned albacore tuna to one 6-ounce serving, and light canned tuna and other lower-mercury fish such as wild salmon and cod to two 6-ounce servings per week. If you don't eat fish, ask your doctor about a fish oil supplement, which contains beneficial omega-3s but is free of the contaminants often found in fish.

Breast milk is about 87 percent water, so be sure to drink plenty of fluids like water and herbal tea. Doctors recommend that nursing moms don't drink more than two to three cups of coffee or caffeinated beverages (no more than 300 milligrams of caffeine) a day. Otherwise, your baby will be bouncing off the wall!

Eat small meals or snacks every two to three hours through-out the day to stave off hunger pangs. Don't let too much time between meals go by; otherwise, you'll be more likely to overin-dulge or reach for fattening foods with little nutritional benefits.

You don't need to avoid spicy, acidic, or gassy foods unless your baby is sensitive to them. Reach for the salsa, beans, and tomatoes! If you expose your baby to a variety of flavors while breastfeeding, your baby may enjoy them later when they start solids.

Indulge once in a while in desserts and special treats, but don't go overboard. One serving is great. Some ideas for healthier des-sert options are:

- Frozen yogurt
- Frozen bananas dipped in chocolate
- Dark chocolate with almonds
- Chocolate avocado pudding
- Black bean brownies
- Banana bread made with quinoa flour
- Peanut butter oatmeal cookies
- Homemade granola bars

How to Increase Your Milk Supply

One of the best ways to increase milk supply is to continue breast-feeding! The more your baby nurses, the more milk your body makes. During the first few weeks of baby's life, the more a baby suckles and stimulates the nipple, the more prolactin is produced, and prolactin stimulates milk production.[24] The emptying of the milk signals your body to increase the milk production.

If you feel like you need to increase your milk supply, there are foods that help promote production. Foods with lactation-pro-moting properties are called lactogenic foods or galactagogues.

Adding lactogenic foods to your diet, along with frequent nursing or pumping, can give your milk supply a boost.

Lactogenic Foods to Add to Your Diet:

- **Oatmeal** has long been recommended as a way for moms to boost their milk supply. Oatmeal has properties that lower cholesterol, maintain a healthy blood pressure, and may also help with lactation.
- **Salmon** contains both EFA and omega-3s, which are highly nutritious and essential for lactating mothers. Opt for steamed, boiled, baked, or even grilled salmon.
- **Spinach** is a good source of calcium, iron, vitamin K, vitamin A, and folate (or folic acid), which is particularly important for women who are pregnant or breastfeeding. Dark leafy green vegetables like spinach also contain phytoestrogens, which are believed to promote breast tissue health and lactation.
- **Carrots** also contain phytoestrogens and are high in beta-carotene and vitamin A, both of which lactating mothers need. Carrots boost lactation and the quality of your milk. A glass of carrot juice with breakfast, carrot sticks with hummus as a snack, or carrots popped in a pot of soup will have wonderful benefits.[25]
- **Legumes** such as chickpeas, lentils, lima beans, or green beans are frequently used lactogenic foods. Hummus, which is traditionally made from chickpeas, tahini, garlic, lemon juice, and olive oil, is a perfect snack for breastfeeding moms. It is a complete protein, and the combination of chickpeas and garlic (another galactagogue) makes this nutrient-dense snack a top choice for nursing moms.
- **Garlic** is well known for boosting lactation in nursing mothers because of its chemical compounds. Toss a few garlic cloves in a stir-fry or soup.

- **Papayas** have been commonly used in Asia as a galact-agogue.[26] It's thought that the enzymes and phytochemicals in papaya may enhance breast tissue as well as improve lactation. Papaya has also been used as a natural sedative. The sedating quality may help you to relax and, at the same time, help with the milk let-down process.

- **Asparagus** is high in fiber, folic acid, and vitamins A, C, and K and contains phytoestrogens. The hormonal effect of phytoestrogens aid in milk production, and high-fiber foods help to maintain a healthy milk supply. Also, asparagus contains tryptophan, an essential amino acid which may stimulate the production of prolactin (a major hormone involved in lactation) and subsequently improve milk supply.

- **Brown rice** is unprocessed rice with just the outermost hull removed. It's a complex carbohydrate, which helps give Mom the energy needed for breastfeeding. It has hormone stimulants that boost lactation. Brown rice is a good source of magnesium, phosphorus, selenium, thiamin, niacin, and vitamin B6 is an excellent source of manganese and protein.

- **Dried apricots** have certain chemicals which balance out the hormone levels in your body, including phytoestrogens, which help to balance the hormones involved in lactation. Apricots are high in fiber, vitamin A, vitamin C, potassium, and calcium. Other calcium-rich dried fruits like figs and dates are thought to help with milk production too.

- **Sweet potato** is a major source of potassium. It has energy-producing carbohydrates, which are needed to fight the fatigue. It also contains vitamins C and B-complex as well as magnesium—a muscle-relaxant mineral. Try cutting sweet potatoes into fries and baking in the oven or mashing them with a touch of almond milk.

Foods That May Cause Issues While Nursing

Breastfeeding moms can enjoy all the foods they normally enjoy; however, it is possible that certain foods can unsettle your baby's tummy. It's thought that dairy products in your diet, such as milk, cheese, and ice cream, can cause colic symptoms. Even other common allergens such as wheat, corn, fish, eggs, or peanuts can cause baby gas.

If you think your baby is reacting to a certain food, try eliminating it from your diet for a week. It might take some guessing, but eliminating a food may help you figure out the cause. Some foods take longer to leave your system. If your baby becomes fussy or develops a rash, diarrhea, or congestion soon after nursing, consult your baby's doctor.

When my son was colicky, I removed cabbage and onions from my diet. Though experts said gassy foods affect only mom's tummy, I found my son and I both felt better. The reason babies have colic is still not clear, but it doesn't hurt to try a change in your diet to help your baby.

If you suspect dairy or meat could be the culprit and need to cut those foods out of your diet completely, you'll need to find other sources of protein. Ask your doctor to refer you to a dietitian who can help you maintain a healthy diet without those foods.

While a tiny amount of what you eat ends up in your milk supply, it's unlikely that a spicy food will affect your baby. In fact, if you are eating a diet rich in flavors and spices, your breast milk may sometimes taste different and baby may be more inclined to try different foods when she starts solids.[27]

If your family has a history of allergies, you might worry about eating foods that can cause a reaction, such as eggs or peanuts. There is no evidence that eating peanuts while breastfeeding makes your baby more likely to develop a peanut allergy. Some research even suggests that continuing to breastfeed while introducing solids may protect your baby against developing food allergies. In fact, new research from the National Institutes of Health recommends that parents introduce peanut-containing foods into the diets of babies as young as four to six months old.[28]

If there is no history of allergy to these foods in the mother's or father's family, you don't need to avoid those foods. If baby has a negative reaction after you've eaten a certain type of food, you can try eliminating that food from your diet for a while.

Foods That May Cause Baby to Have a Reaction

- **Caffeine:** I know; you can't live without coffee or tea, especially those first three months! While you may have a cup or two, you don't want to overdo it. That extra-large takeout coffee will likely keep your baby awake during naptime. Don't forget that chocolate also has caffeine—as well as a laxative effect! If baby becomes fussy or has a runny poop after a chocolate binge, you may have to cut back or eliminate chocolate completely.
- **Dairy:** Dairy is one of the most common problem foods for breastfed babies. If your baby is especially fussy after nursing, has trouble sleeping, or has eczema or other skin issues, dairy products may be the cause. Try eliminating dairy from your diet to see if your baby improves.
- **Alcohol:** A glass of wine with dinner is tempting! Alcohol does go into your breast milk and will be taken in by your baby when you are nursing. According to the American Academy of Pediatrics, excessive or regular drinking is discouraged during breastfeeding. An occasional celebratory single, small alcoholic drink is acceptable, but the AAP and other experts suggest that mothers wait about two hours before resuming breastfeeding.[29]

- **Garlic:** While garlic may help boost lactation in nursing mothers, some babies may not like the taste of garlic, which can get into your milk! If you find that baby is reluctant to nurse, it could be the garlic.
- **Wheat:** Does your baby have bloody stools? Fussiness and a painful tummy can signify wheat and gluten intolerance. The best way to determine if wheat is an issue is to follow an elimination diet. You can choose to eliminate all common problem-causing foods and then slowly start reintroducing them one at a time to determine which food is the cause. Keep a journal so you can go back and pinpoint what triggers a reaction.
- **Citrus:** Since your baby's tummy is still immature, some of the compounds in citrus fruits can be irritating. Consuming citrus fruits and juices can cause baby to be fussy, spit up, or have a diaper rash. Go easy on the orange juice and lemon zest for a few days and see if baby improves.

To determine links between your diet and your baby's behavior, keep a food diary. List everything you eat and drink along with notes about how your baby reacts—if at all. If removing a food or drink from your diet has no impact on your baby's fussiness, add it back into your diet and consider other culprits. If you think your baby is reacting to a certain food but you can't seem to figure out what is bothering him, talk to your doctor.

If you do breastfeed, you'll see the wonderful benefits both for baby and you too! While you may encounter some difficulties along the way, you'll see that the rewards are worth it. Keep in mind that although you don't need to eat twice the calories, you are still eating for two, so explore what foods are best and eat well.

Chapter Six

CHOOSING BOTTLE

Research shows that *breast is best*, as breast milk contains all the vitamins and nutrients your baby needs in the first six months of life and is packed with disease-fighting substances that protect your baby from illness. However, breastfeeding doesn't work for all women due to various circumstances, including medical reasons and personal choices. If breastfeeding doesn't work for you, *fed is best*. This term was coined by the Fed Is Best Foundation, which believes that babies should never go hungry and mothers should be supported in choosing safe feeding options for their babies, whether breast milk, formula, or a combination of both.[30]

Some new moms decide to breastfeed while supplementing with formula because they find that is the best choice for their family and their lifestyle. The decision to breastfeed or formula-feed your baby (or both!) is a personal one and must be based on a woman's lifestyle, comfort level, and medical situation. For mothers who are unable to breastfeed or who decide not to, infant formula provides babies with the nutrients they need to grow and thrive. It's crucial for mom to be equipped with research and be well educated before making this personal decision.

Reasons Moms Choose to Bottle-Feed

You Feel You're Not Producing Enough Milk

If you feel something isn't right—if your baby isn't producing enough wet diapers, isn't satisfied after a feeding, or is constantly crying after a feeding or if you suspect you aren't producing enough milk—push to have your voice heard. If you feel you are being pressured to avoid supplementation to alleviate your child's hunger, talk to your doctor, pediatrician, and/or the hospital administrator.

One in five newborns may need supplemented milk, especially babies of first-time mothers who have delayed onset of copious milk production, according to the Fed Is Best Foundation.[31] Twenty-two percent of mothers have been found to have a delay in copious milk production, which means there is a lag from the time of birth to when enough milk *comes in* to completely support her baby's needs.[32]

However, in another study, it was found that up to 50 percent of women report that they perceive their milk supply to be insufficient while only about 5 percent of women suffer from a physiologically insufficient supply.[33] This means that many women perceive they are not producing enough milk and then supplement breastfeeding with formula, which then reduces the demand for breast milk and decreases their supply.

When your baby is given formula supplements, baby is drinking less from the breast, so the breasts respond by making less milk. If supplementation is necessary, pumping as well as breast-feeding can help to increase milk production. Now baby is fed, and, when milk supply is established, Mom can choose to provide all or most of baby's feedings with breast milk, or Mom may decide formula works best. It really must be about feeding baby in a way that works best for Mom and baby.

If supplementing and pumping does not increase milk supply, know that fed is best. Consult with your doctor or pediatrician and feel confident that formula is best for you and your baby. Plenty of well-adjusted adults have been raised on formula—including me!

The Mechanics Are Just Not Working

There are several reasons why breast milk won't come in or a mom's milk supply just can't reach sweet baby's tummy:

Labor

A long labor, use of labor medications, and having a C-section can all contribute to milk supply delay or shortage. Mothers who received labor pain medications—whether spinal/epidural agents or other pain-relief medications like Demerol during a vaginal delivery or C-section—were more likely to report delayed onset of lactation.

Flat or Inverted Nipples

Flat or inverted nipples can also be an issue. How do you know? Here's the fun part—test to see whether your nipples are really flat or inverted! Do the simple "pinch" test: hold your breast at the edge of the areola between your thumb and index finger. Press in gently but firmly about an inch behind your nipple. If your nipple protrudes, you're good to go. If it does not protrude or become erect, it is considered flat. If it retracts or disappears, it is truly inverted.

While one breast might be flat or inverted, the other might be just fine. Or you may have one nipple that protrudes more than the other. It's not unusual for a mother to produce more milk from one breast than the other. I remember one boob would gush milk while the other would be a mere trickle.

Check with a lactation expert, as there are things you can do if you still want to nurse. They make nipple shields, which work for many women to create a better nipple shape for latching. They are not fun but may allow you to nurse if you wish to try. Sometimes even if you weren't able to nurse with your first child, you may be able to with a subsequent child.

Medical Issues

Another reason for low milk supply is baby's health at birth. Hopefully baby is born healthy and mom is healthy, but if there is a medical issue and baby needs to be separated from mom, he may be given formula. If your baby is in the neonatal intensive care unit, you may need to adjust your plans and use a combination of breast milk and formula. Bottle-feeding and nursing/pumping in a way that works best for you and your baby will be your best option. Many premature babies need to save energy for other things— growing and nursing uses a lot of energy.

Baby's Tongue or Palate

Baby could have a tongue-tie; the thin membrane of tissue at the bottom of his mouth is holding the baby's tongue too tightly so that he's not able to use it properly to extract the milk. Check to see if your baby is able to stick his tongue out over his bottom lip. Baby's tongue should also be touching the roof of his mouth when he cries. If your baby is tongue-tied, the membrane can be clipped by a doctor, and the baby's ability to breastfeed will improve quickly. A cleft lip and cleft palate may also be the cause. If baby isn't feeding well, check with an expert or your doctor.

Postpartum Depression

Women who have postpartum depression may find they have difficulties breastfeeding, have a low sense of self-efficacy, and breastfeed for a shorter period. If you're becoming increasingly frustrated and stressed, the pressure of breastfeeding may worsen your depression symptoms. Talk to a professional to address both issues. Remember: fed is always best.

Mom Needs to Return to Work or School

If you breastfeed but plan to switch to formula once you're back at work, pumping can seem stressful. It can also be a logistical challenge: when and where to pump, how often, where to store the milk, etc. If you want to try both breast and bottle while at work, have your baby drink formula during the day but nurse before you leave for work and after you return home from work. Your baby will still benefit, and you'll both enjoy the bonding time. Your body will adapt to the change as well. Or you can try pumping once or twice while at work and then only offer from the breast when you're home.

If you decided to exclusively formula-feed, then you'll need to wean slowly. A few weeks before your maternity leave ends, start pumping once or twice during the day and give your baby a bottle instead of nursing him. This will help your midday supply start to diminish so that you can avoid painful engorgement at work. At first you can offer a mix of formula and breast milk and see if baby responds to it. If baby doesn't reject the bottle, you're in luck!

Some babies can become picky by three months; some might take a bottle while others refuse it. Some babies prefer bottles because they can get more milk in a shorter time and with less work. But if you want to continue offering both breast and formula, begin slowly with supplementing and keep portion size small. Start with two ounces in a four-ounce bottle, with slow-flow nipples—which are harder work for the baby—mimicking the breast.

Tips for Bottle Feeding

You'll quickly find that bottle-feeding takes some organizing and planning. You'll need to make sure you have formula and all the necessary supplies, like bottles and nipples, clean and ready to go when baby is hungry. Especially the first few weeks with baby eating often, parents can quickly become overwhelmed if they're not prepared!

The convenience of a bottle is obvious; any parent or caregiver can prepare and feed the baby a bottle at any time (this is also true for women who pump and store their breast milk). Assign the task to Dad or your mother- or father-in-law so they can bond. Use a nursing pillow to prop baby up, and snuggle baby close, keeping that eye contact as you feed! Be sure to keep bottle angled so that baby is not sucking air.

There are three types of formula: ready-to-feed, concentrated liquid, and powdered. To keep your baby safe, powdered formula must be prepared exactly as listed on the container. Ready-to-feed and concentrated liquid formulas do not have any bacteria and are sterile until they are opened. Powdered formula is the least expensive, followed by concentrated, with ready-to-feed being the most expensive.

Most formula available today has cow's milk as the main ingredient. But there are other types, including soy and hypoallergenic formulas and specialty formulas that are gentle for babies' tummies to consider. Talk to your doctor about the type of formula that is best for your baby. If you're new to bottle-feeding, you might want to select one brand's starter kit, which will come in two sizes: four-ounce bottles geared towards newborns, who eat less, and larger eight-ounce bottles for older babies. Kits may also come with various-size nipples: slow, medium, and fast flow for older babies.

You may opt for glass bottles, which are sturdy and long lasting but also heavy, typically more expensive, and can shatter. Or you can choose plastic bottles, which are lightweight and virtually unbreakable but can wear out faster. Plastic bottles are now required to be free of a chemical called bisphenol A (BPA). I don't recommend picking up bottles secondhand, as they may contain BPA.

The best way to warm your baby's bottle is to put it in a cup of warm water, or you may want to use a bottle warmer, which will heat the formula to just the right temperature. Test the milk on your wrist to make sure it isn't too hot first. Do not microwave your baby's bottle, as the milk can heat unevenly and potentially burn your baby's mouth and throat.

Because formula is less digestible than breast milk, formula-fed babies usually need to eat less often than breastfed babies. On the downside, formula-fed babies may have more gas and firmer bowel movements than breastfed babies. If you don't want that precious milk regurgitated onto your furniture, be sure to burp your baby well. This helps painful gas bubbles that often accumulate in baby's belly since their digestive system is still so delicate. This is something Dad can get involved with as well.

If you plan to be away for less than a couple of hours, you can bring prepared formula in an insulated bag or cooler with an ice pack. But if you plan to be away from home for longer than two hours, the best option is to bring unopened ready-to-feed formula with you.

All prepared formula should be fed immediately or refrigerated and fed to your baby within twenty-four hours. Throw away any open ready-to-feed or concentrated formula after forty-eight hours. Discard any prepared or ready-to-feed formula that's been sitting out after one hour.

You can pre-make and refrigerate bottles in the morning; if you know your baby eats every three to four hours, for instance, you can make six to eight bottles to last you all day. Now all you have to do is warm and shake gently.

Guilt in Deciding on a Bottle

Some mothers worry that if they don't breastfeed, they won't bond with their baby. But the truth is, you can create a special bond with your baby no matter how baby is fed. If you wanted to breastfeed but then decided not to or are forced to give it up, you may feel upset and disappointed.

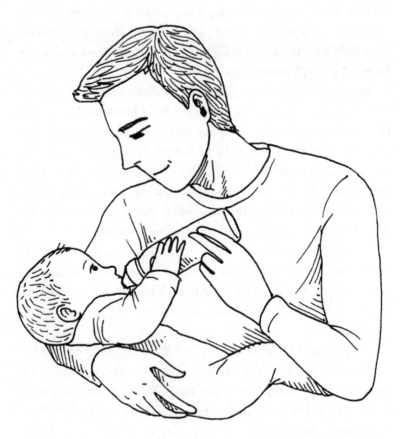

For many new moms, the struggle is very real, and after trying to breastfeed unsuccessfully, they feel they have to quit. If you are feeling this way, weigh the pros and cons before making a decision. If you are experiencing breastfeeding issues, consult your doctor.

Women who have difficulty with breastfeeding often turn to lactation consultants, whose mantra is "breast is best." They'll encourage you through the bleeding nipples, the poor milk production, and the immense frustration to get it right. For some women, a little guidance from an expert can help, while for others, it further increases the frustration. They may feel intense pressure to breastfeed and fear being judged if they bottle-feed their babies.

The decision to bottle-feed can be an excruciating one! I know many moms who have felt conflicted by the choice to stop nursing because of the challenges they faced. They felt so much guilt for choosing to feed their babies formula.

While breastfeeding has many benefits, if nursing causes you anxiety or worry and impedes your mental well-being, then you need to reconsider. Breastfeeding should not make you miserable! A happy mom is also important to baby! You can still experience the closeness of breastfeeding by cuddling your baby against your warm skin while you bottle-feed.

You'll come to realize that breastfeeding or bottle-feeding doesn't measure your success as a mother. What matters most is that your baby is growing and well-fed and you are happy and thriving as well.

Mom to Mom

I chose to bottle-feed from the beginning. I did not feel any pressure at all from the hospital. They gave me a bottle right away to feed. The only time I was challenged regarding breastfeeding versus bottle-feeding was when I went to Walmart to exchange formulas. The woman at the return counter commented that I wouldn't need to exchange anything if I breastfed my baby. I was shocked, but another mom came to the rescue and told her off. I thought that was super nice for another mom to come to my defense.
—Melissa Thompson

When I was pregnant, I thought breastfeeding would be so easy and natural. I was wrong—so wrong. After a difficult birth, I was exhausted and then had to deal with a tongue-tied baby who wouldn't and couldn't latch. The thickest tongue the pediatrician had ever seen. After weeks at the breastfeeding clinic, giving gradual cuts to release it, feeding tubes, destroyed nipples, and sleepless nights, I ended up with PPD—some dark days for me. We went to formula and never looked back. I realized that it was okay—happy mommy meant happy baby. My baby bonded with my husband as he could feed baby too, and we all flourished. Fast forward three years, and I have a new baby. In my head, I had said I'm not going to beat myself up this time around. If breastfeeding works, great. *Well, I got a five-week-early baby who had a lazy suck and didn't want to latch again. I pumped for two months until I felt it was enough and got out the bottles again. It went much smoother this time around, and I kept my PPD at bay because I was in more control. Happy mommy means happy babies.*
—Caroline Dawn

I formula-fed my daughter; I tried to breastfeed and pump for a couple weeks, but my milk wasn't coming in, and it made me frustrated. I was tired and emotional and felt that most of my day was trying to get milk out. I decided to stop trying and formula-feed. In my opinion, it was the best decision we made. I had a very happy, healthy baby. She never was once sick in her first year on the earth and slept through the night at ten weeks. Of course, you feel pressure to breastfeed, but it's my baby and my choice. I'm currently twenty-three weeks pregnant with number two, and I'll give breastfeeding a try again, but I will be fine to formula-feed if that works best. —Katie Taylor

Chapter Seven

MOM'S FIRST OUTINGS

Some new moms feel stir crazy and take the baby out almost immediately after arriving home. They feel they need to get out and chat with other adults. Other new moms prefer the comfort and safety of staying home those first few weeks after baby is born. Often moms need more time to recover and aren't feeling well enough or comfortable yet to go out. A difficult childbirth, a preemie, or just feeling anxious and nervous about going out are all valid reasons to hunker down and stay put. I felt like I was becoming too comfortable in my cozy cocoon. I think the longer I waited to go out, the more anxious about it I became. I was a little scared to venture out with my baby!

When it comes to your first outing, you must do what feels comfortable for you. If you don't feel ready to venture out yet, don't. The time will come eventually! And those first doctor's appointments will force you out if the need for sustenance or fresh air did not already get you out and about.

When to Take Baby Out

Older relatives may frighten you by saying that taking baby out can be dangerous or that it isn't proper for a new mother to take baby out in busy public places. At the same time, you'll also see some newborn babies traveling at the mall or the grocery store. There is no correct medical answer as to when baby can first go out.

During the first six to eight weeks, the baby's immune system is still developing, making him susceptible to germs. Babies are born with some of their mom's immunities in place, and breast-feeding is important to help keep baby's immune system strong. Minimizing your child's exposure to illness will give him a chance to get his immune system up and running rather than having baby need to fight off something he's not ready to handle. Newborns aren't fully armed to tackle every germ out there, and the last thing you want is for your infant to get sick. If your baby has any health issues or concerns, speak to baby's doctor before heading out.

When you do go out, make sure that people wash their hands with soap and water before handling your baby. Also, avoid any-one who is sick or recovering from illness. While many experts say it's perfectly fine to take your newborn out of the house, you may wish to avoid busy places like the supermarket, shopping mall, or other crowded places. Instead, go for a walk. The outdoors are less germy than indoors. Fresh air and a little sunshine are great for both of you!

Taking Newborn Out

Taking baby out may seem daunting for new mothers. There is so much to remember! No longer can you throw on a jacket, grab your purse, and hop into your car. With a baby, you'll feel you need to bring along everything including the kitchen sink!

When you have an infant in tow, being organized can make your outings much easier and more enjoyable. Prepare a diaper or baby bag with all of the essentials that you or baby may need on your outings. Here are some of the things you might need while you're out and about with baby:

- Diapers and wipes
- Changing pad
- Diaper cream or ointment
- Baby blanket
- Change of clothing
- Pacifiers
- Burping/feeding blanket
- Sun hat and baby sunscreen
- Nursing cover and nursing pads
- Bottle and formula or breast milk
- Sterile water
- Stroller rain cover
- Sun UV ray cover
- Parenting/baby book
- Baby toys

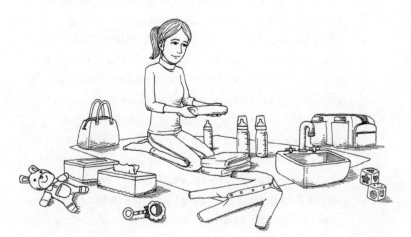

It may seem like a lot of items to lug around, but you can also keep some of these items readily available in your diaper bag and in a basket in the trunk of your car. It is a good idea to keep an extra infant outfit, diapers, and wipes in the car at all times in case of emergencies . . . and an extra top for you too—new babies have so many options for destroying mom's outfit.

You will likely forget something at one point or another! Pregnancy brain lasts longer than pregnancy, just so you're aware . . . well into the first year of motherhood. Keeping written lists or notes around the house or using an app on your cell phone can help keep you organized.

Having the essentials handy will put you at ease, but you may still feel nervous when heading out. Try these tips to help make you feel more prepared for your first outing.

- Layer baby's clothing, unless the temperature is over 75 degrees Fahrenheit. Your baby will need several layers of clothing to keep warm. You can dress baby in an undershirt and diaper, covered by pajamas or a dressing gown, and then wrap her in a receiving blanket. For an extra layer, a wearable blanket sleeper or sleep sack is a safe layer of warmth. You can tuck a cozy blanket over her once she's buckled into her car seat—bulky outerwear shouldn't be worn under her harness.

- In hot weather (over 75 degrees Fahrenheit), baby can wear one layer. A good rule of thumb is to dress the baby in one more layer of clothing than you are wearing to be comfortable in the same environment.

- If you need to do a diaper change while you're out, choose clothing that can be removed easily. A sleeper or onesie with snaps all the way up the legs is so much easier than tights and fluffy dresses (for you and baby, too).

- For the first outing, try going on a walk in the neighborhood or running a quick errand. If you're already feeling comfortable, then stay out longer. Feed and change baby right before you go out. That way, you know you'll have a couple of hours before the next feeding and diaper change.

- Give yourself enough time to be ready. If you need to be somewhere at 10:00 a.m., give yourself at least a half hour before heading out to prepare. It will take longer than you think! I would plan and organize myself so I'd have enough time before heading out, yet I'd still manage to be late. Baby may want to nurse longer or have a wet diaper and then, right after changing, have a poop explosion! One time, I had just finished getting my son ready when all of a sudden, he pooped his pants with such a force, the explosion went through his onesie and sleeper and all the way up his back! There goes another fifteen minutes trying to clean him up again!

- Maybe it was just my uncoordinated self, but I would often spend a few minutes trying to figure out how to close baby's stroller. The people at the baby store made it look so easy! I'd be flustered trying to figure out all these latches, and sometimes it would jam when I tried to close it. There were times when I'd be stuffing the stroller—unfolded—into the trunk of my van because I lost patience trying to figure it out!

- Think about how you may handle certain situations where you're going. For example, will there be baby changing facilities there? If you prefer privacy, is there a separate place to nurse? Is there somewhere to warm milk if needed? It's helpful to keep these things in mind so you're prepared if a situation arises. Because I was anxious, I didn't feel comfortable nursing in public right away. At the time, they didn't have as many nursing stations as they do nowadays, so when baby was hungry,

I would panic to find a quiet spot to feed him. In hindsight, I would've just popped out my breast right there (with a cover, though, for my comfort) and fed baby instantly. When possible, choose baby-friendly venues where you know there will be amenities for moms with infants.

- Go early or late to avoid the crowds. You don't want to be stuck in traffic or waiting in lines. Don't overdo your outing. Plan a trip lasting no more than two hours, at least the first time, so you can see how comfortable you are with baby.

I remember really pushing one of our outings; it was past the two-hour mark, I was waiting in a long line, and the baby started crying nonstop. There have been many times where I've ended up leaving a store to calm baby down. Once, I even left a cart of groceries behind because baby was crying uncontrollably. Sometimes kind shoppers have invited me to cut the line, while other times, I've simply asked, "Would you mind if I go ahead of you?" Usually the wails coming from the stroller help.

How to Deal with Strangers

You're taking your baby out for a walk in the city. But your plan doesn't go as well as you thought! As you're trying to enjoy a stroll, the sidewalks are crowded with people, a few passersby are smoking, and then it suddenly begins to rain. You run into a coffee shop for cover. But then the baby admirers come over to see your baby. One is sneezing; the other is coughing! What do you do?

If baby is sleeping, put a privacy cover over the top of baby's stroller. These breathable covers keep the air circulating but also prevent admirers ogling.

Once, I took my baby to do some shopping, and an older woman walked up to us and told us how cute my baby was. Before

I could even utter a "Thank you," she had grabbed his hand. I was a little nervous, because the only thing I could think of was GERMS! But I know the lady meant well, and seeing my baby probably made her morning a little brighter. As soon as she left, I reached into my diaper bag and grabbed a wipe to clean his hands.

If strangers are trying to get too close, trying to touch or pick up baby, you can politely say, "I'm sorry; I know you mean well, but my baby is very young and susceptible to germs," or, "Oh, baby is susceptible to germs, so we shouldn't be touching him if hands aren't clean," or, even more direct and simple, "Please don't touch my baby." All these work great. Don't be afraid to speak up. Strangers think it's okay to touch a baby's hand or even their cheeks! But it's not cool, even if they mean well.

If the person insists, be polite and honest. "I'm not comfortable with people touching my child, so please don't. He can get sick." Say it with a smile so the stranger realizes you're being a protective mom and not trying to be rude. You can also tell people that your baby doesn't respond well to strangers and that she has stranger anxiety. "She'll start crying if anyone she doesn't know touches her" might work to get people to back off. If the stranger persists, be firm. This is your baby, not a piece of fruit at the grocery store.

If you see someone eyeing baby and you're pretty sure they are about to approach you, run! You can swivel the stroller and head in the opposite direction. You can also place a breathable cover over baby's stroller—this usually acts as a good deterrent. You may have the odd bold person lifting up the netting or cover and still reaching for baby, but this extra layer will give you time to tell the stranger that touching your baby is not okay.

Outing Ideas

Getting out of the house is a nice way to break up your day. When you're up to it, here are some ideas to help lift your spirits and expose baby to new surroundings.

- Go for a car ride. Don't drive, however, if you are taking prescription pain relievers. Most doctors will advise waiting three to six weeks if you have had a C-section, are anemic, or have had a painful episiotomy. There are many times I've gone through a coffee drive-thru and then taken a nice drive in the country. I'll put the music on (not too loud) and enjoy the landscape while baby usually falls asleep.

- Check with your local library to see if they have any programs for new moms and babies, like a Mother Goose type of class. You can also visit a bookstore and peruse the baby book section or find a great mystery for you and baby. Entertain yourself and let baby hear the flow of language. It's all good!

- Check with your La Leche League chapter for a mother-to-mother breastfeeding support group in your area.

- After your doctor gives you the all clear, check out a mommy-and-baby fitness class, dance class, or yoga class. It'll be fun to meet other moms in your area while getting some exercise. You and baby can have fun learning to salsa!

- A change of scenery in a cozy coffee shop may just be enough to make you feel refreshed. Often just being around other people rather than your four walls can do wonders!

- Go for a stroller walk. But when you do, take it easy at first—don't overdo it. Listen to your body for cues that you're overexerting yourself. Most doctors recommend waiting until your six-week postpartum checkup to begin fitness walks.

- Join a local mom's group for outings with other moms. Check your mall to see if they have a group stroller walk for new moms. Facebook has a ton of local mom groups that often arrange get-togethers with other new moms. You can also check Meetups.com for local mom groups!

No matter what you choose to do, meeting new moms and getting out with baby or just going solo will do wonders!

Mom to Mom

Don't put pressure on yourself for your first outing to be perfect, because it won't be. Between the botched first attempt at nursing in public to the crying right as you're checking out, it can be overwhelming. If you expect too much, you might be disappointed. Just plan a small outing so you can experience success and build your confidence. Don't hesitate to ask a fellow parent to borrow a wipe or an extra set of hands; we're in it together! —Monica Bertenshaw

Start small and carry a big bag . . . and pack that bag with something for every eventuality that might occur with the baby plus an extra shirt for you. —Megan Houston

If you second-guess packing something: JUST PACK IT! If you don't, you'll definitely need it! Keep your outing short. I was feeling pretty good and tried to go shopping six days after my son was born. After fifteen minutes, I could barely walk anymore; I was so sore down there! —Jacklyn De Ciccio

Double the diapers, double the wipes . . . oh, and a few plastic bags. —Chriss Bickers

Bring extra baby clothes. Plastic bags and wet bags (waterproof fabric bags with cute designs) are a big must! Time your feedings so your baby is not hungry if you're stuck in traffic. Make sure the restaurants or places you go to are baby friendly, like having baby stations. I went to a few places where washrooms were not built to code and I had to improvise or change baby in the car. A baby carrier is super useful when you're shopping alone or when you have no help so your arms are free. Always have instant ready-to-go formula with a one-time-use nipple in the bag just in case, because you never know! Don't be lazy and think you can carry the car seat to the breast clinic or a place that you have never explored . . . take a minute and take the stroller out . . . because that baby car seat is super heavy when you are wandering around for more than ten min-utes! —Garman Wong

I would say pack the house, but since you can't, bring some tiny comforts from home: soother, blankie, stuffy, etc. Bring lots of diapers and wipes, a change of clothes for baby AND for YOU; you will be barfed on, or you will leak, and you know what, we usually pack lots for baby and never think of ourselves, but WE need things too! —Alessia Giacomi

Don't plan to stay out too long, and if possible, bring some-one with you. —Megan Smith

My advice: get out! It doesn't matter what season it is, what atrocities your body has been through, how tired you are, how dirty you feel, how alone you are, how small your baby is . . . get out. Get out that first day (even if you just walk to the end of the driveway) and every day. —Kim Madore

My advice for the first outing is to keep it short and make sure you don't have to be somewhere at a scheduled time. Get everything ready to go and THEN do your last feeding and head out. For me, the early days of breastfeeding were challenging and I couldn't have managed doing it in pub-lic, so our outings were scheduled in between feedings. And yes, bring lots of extra clothes . . . for baby AND yourself! —Janelle Dayman

Chapter Eight

DOCTOR APPOINTMENTS

Baby's First Doctor Visit

The first few outings you'll have with baby are likely going to be to and from the doctor's office. The American Academy of Pediatrics (AAP) recommends babies get checkups at birth, three to five days after birth, and then at month one, two, four, six, nine, and twelve. Your pediatrician or family doctor's schedule may be slightly different.

Baby's first appointment will come up quicker than you think! Those first weeks feel like a blur of nighttime feeding, diapers and more diapers, and sweet napping moments (I am referring to when *you* get to sleep!). Before you have a chance to blink, it's time for a trip to the doctor. It's helpful to bring someone with you the first time to help with the baby so you have an extra pair of hands while you ask the doctor questions. I found it helpful to go prepared with a list of questions and a pen to jot down any answers as well as the baby's weight and height.

Our pediatrician's office was always busy, and the typical wait to see him was at least an hour. Be prepared to fill out some forms while you wait. Bring paperwork from the hospital, including baby's discharge weight as well as information about baby's birth. Bring your own medical history too.

I learned quickly that having a well-stocked diaper bag came in handy. You'll also need a blanket to keep baby warm while you wait; you'll have to undress baby for the physical examination. The nurse will weigh and measure baby, and doctor will check baby from head to toe. While you wait for the doctor to come and see baby, it is very possible for baby to decide *right then* to pee or poop on the examination table or while he's wrapped in a blanket in your arms! It's a good idea to keep a clean diaper on baby while you wait.

You will soon learn how baby is growing. Is she back up to birth weight? Are her muscle tone and skin normal? Baby's heart, lungs, belly, eyes, mouth, ears, legs, and even her sweet bum will all get a check.

The doctor will feel baby's head, checking the fontanel, the two soft spots on baby's skull which allow for baby's brain to develop and head to grow. The softs spots can also show that baby is properly hydrated. Doc will roll baby's hips to ensure baby's joints are where they should be and check baby's reflexes to make sure she is responsive and has proper reflexive actions. The doctor will examine the umbilical cord, press the skin along the side of baby's groin, and check baby's genitalia.

The doctor will ask how often baby is eating, how long your breast-feeding sessions take, and if there are any latching issues. If you're formula-feeding, he'll ask how much, how often, and what type of formula. He'll also ask how many times you change baby's diaper per day to ensure baby is digesting and absorbing nutrients well.

Lastly, the doctor may ask about sleeping patterns and sleep safety, making sure baby is sleeping on her back. Doc may ask you if you're also getting enough sleep . . . you may laugh right in their face at this question! This is the best time to discuss any questions about baby's sleeping and eating and even your milk supply.

I was impressed by my pediatrician's skill in checking all those wiggling body parts so quickly before baby began to fuss. Newborns will want to be in your arms for comfort. When baby is older, soft, colorful, and noisy toys help keep baby distracted—especially during vaccinations.

Vaccinations have tiny amounts of weakened or inactivated viruses and bacteria (known as antigens) that trigger the immune system to create antibodies that fight against them. These antibodies are prepared to attack if the body is exposed to those viruses or bacteria again.

No parent looks forward to their baby's vaccinations. You may dread those immunizations because, oh my gosh, needles. But remember that vaccinating your child will build his immune system to fight off life-threatening diseases. While there has been much controversy and discussion surrounding vaccinations, the medical consensus is that they are safe and efficient and that the benefits far outweigh the risks.

The combination of cuddling and feeding or sucking, along with anesthetic cream on the injection site before baby is given a vaccine, will help alleviate pain, more so than distracting your baby with a favorite toy or a song.[34] To help reduce the pain of needles and comfort baby, hold him on your lap while you nurse or give a bottle. Hugs plus something sweet and satisfying actually reduces pain! (There must be some way to apply this during labor!)

If you're not breastfeeding or don't want to during shots, your pediatrician may have some sucrose solution on hand, or you can make your own at home by mixing one teaspoon of table sugar with two teaspoons of clean water. Give to your baby on a pacifier or through a dropper a minute before the needle. Talk to your doctor about the anesthetic cream.

My babies didn't cry for more than about twenty seconds after shots. I think I cried longer than they did! It's common for babies to have a mild fever and be fussier than usual for a day or two after receiving vaccines, which simply means that your child is having an appropriate immune response to the vaccine. You'll want to give your baby lots of hugs and cuddles, as the injection site might be a bit sore. Your baby may even experience a slight loss of appetite. But if baby is crying inconsolably for more than three hours or develops a high fever, seizures, swelling of the face, or limpness, get immediate medical help.

Mom's First Doctor Visit

You also have to get a checkup around six weeks after giving birth. Your postpartum checkup is an ideal opportunity for you to consult your doctor about any concerns you have following the birth of your baby and to see how you're healing after delivery.

Your doctor will give you a pelvic exam to make sure that your uterus has returned to its pre-pregnancy size. Your doctor will also feel your ovaries for growths and perform a Pap smear to check for abnormal cervical cells. I felt super anxious about the six-week checkup because the last thing I wanted was anything probing down there! After an episiotomy with my first and tearing with my second, healing took longer than I anticipated. Though I was dreading the whole thing, it went just fine. And I was reassured that all was well.

If you bring your baby to this appointment, make sure to have someone with you while you're being examined. Or, if you don't have someone with you, having a car seat or stroller for baby to sit in while the exam is being performed will be helpful. For my first visit, I brought baby with me; I didn't want to be without him for a few hours! I figured I'd have to venture out on my own with baby at some point, and the doctor's office was a good practice run. It went smoother than I anticipated; I breastfed in the waiting room and used an empty office to change baby. My doctor was also thrilled to see the baby she helped bring into the world!

If you've had a C-section, you'll probably have a preliminary incision checkup at around two weeks and another at six weeks. You may still feel numbness around the site of the incision, but sensation should gradually return as the nerve endings renew themselves. If you had a vaginal delivery and suffered a tear or episiotomy, the doctor will want to check the incision to ensure that it's healing well.

Your doctor may check your abdomen to see if the muscles are returning to normal since occasionally the abdominal muscles separate after birth, known as diastasis recti. If the muscles are more than four fingers apart, you may be referred to a physical therapist. Pilates and core conditioning exercises can help, and your doctor may talk to you about these exercises.

Backaches can be a problem after baby's birth too. The pregnancy hormone relaxin, which softens muscles and ligaments in preparation for childbirth, remains in the body for about four months after baby arrives. Your doctor may talk to you about your posture, how you're carrying or feeding your baby, and the benefits of exercise.

Incontinence is quite common after childbirth, so don't feel embarrassed to mention this to your doctor. He or she may encourage you to do Kegel exercises, and if the problem persists, you may be referred to a physical therapist for bladder-training exercises. I promise—you will be glad to get help on this one.

Your doctor may also assess your emotional state as well to check for postpartum depression symptoms. If you're feeling overwhelmed, your doctor may be able to put you in touch with some support services to help you through this period (see Chapter 9). Speak up if you feel overly sad or anxious. PPD is very treatable, whether you opt for traditional medicine or a holistic approach.

If all is well with your health and well-being, your doctor will likely give the all-clear to resume regular activity . . . and that also means having sex again. Your doctor will ask you what your plans are for contraception and discuss birth control options. It is quite possible to become pregnant right after coming home from the hospital . . . you may not want a surprise so quickly after giving birth!

Have a list of questions ready. Answers from your doctor will help you make the transition to motherhood smoothly.

The first few outings to the doctor's office will be good practice for when you're ready to venture out with baby to the grocery store, to the shopping mall, or to visit friends. You'll find you'll have gained a new sense of confidence as a mom and you will be on track in caring for yourself and your little one!

Chapter Nine

BABY BLUES WHO? POSTPARTUM IS KILLER

You're home and sitting on bags of frozen peas, wondering where all the good daytime dramas like *Santa Barbara*, *As The World Turns*, and *Another World* went. That first week of being home with baby is daunting. It's just you, *LIVE with Kelly and Ryan*, and your little baby who relies on you for everything. Bringing baby home and beginning this new chapter of my life was a huge change for me. I was pretty good at going to work and taking care of myself and hubby, but mommy-and-me time 24/7 was quite a transition.

My mom lives close by, and having her near really helped. She'd come and visit every day and bring me food, which is a godsend when your milk comes in. I was constantly hungry and wanting nutritious meals. But when you have stitches and are feeding every ninety minutes, you really don't have time to cook. I was thankful for those bowls of chicken soup she sent my way. Thinking back to those first few weeks, those hot, homemade meals were a lifesaver.

My sister was also in town, so she came over, and we talked and laughed together. Having her around for company was wonderful, but once she left, I felt really sad. The blues kicked in, and I was very emotional. When I held my baby, I felt intense love and pride, but it was mixed with frustration and concern. As I sat breastfeeding, I would become weepy. I had immense and profound love for this little human being who was a part of me. At the same time, the overwhelming feeling of responsibility was terrifying. Could I be a good mother? How could a new mother, who is supposed to feel so much joy and love, have feelings of intense sadness? I'm home with my happy, healthy baby, so why do I feel so horrible?

After several weeks had passed, I realized that the blues weren't quite disappearing. Instead, I was feeling more and more weepy, crying for no reason, and feeling isolated. I felt overwhelmed with emotion . . . first, pride and joy, but then feelings of loneliness. I felt huge pressure to instantly become this self-sufficient, amazing mom who could breastfeed on demand, entertain people who wanted to come over and see the baby, and look like a real person when I still had the post-pregnancy belly and a bra stuffed with pads. All I really wanted to do was sleep. I couldn't have cared less about family members, let alone friends. Having to put out appetizers or dessert and serve them ginger ale and coffee was not helping me. I wanted everyone to just go away.

I couldn't even begin to think about making meals—it was like I was plucked away from my regular routine and put on a foreign planet without any knowledge or understanding of what was happening around me. I was on Mars gasping for air. I couldn't function, let alone get to feeling somewhat normal.

What Is the Difference Between the Baby Blues and Postpartum Depression?

What does it feel like to have the baby blues, postpartum depression, or postpartum anxiety? What are the signs or symptoms? How do you know when you have it?

The baby blues affects many new mothers in the first few days after giving birth. While not all moms experience the blues, some feel weepy, irritable, tired, and/or stressed due to the hormonal changes in her body. Hey—you just made a human; there are some side effects!

Postpartum depression (PPD), unlike the baby blues, is an illness and is unlikely to disappear without treatment. PPD is very common. A 2013 study in *JAMA Psychiatry* says one of every seven mothers, or 14 percent, will get PPD.[35]

Baby Blues Symptoms

Knowing the difference between the baby blues and postpartum depression is important. The American Pregnancy Association lists the signs and symptoms of baby blues, which last only a few days to a week or two after your baby is born.

Symptoms may include:
- Anxiety
- Sadness
- Weepiness or crying for no apparent reason
- Irritability
- Impatience
- Restlessness
- Fatigue
- Insomnia
- Mood swings
- Reduced concentration[36]

Baby blues affects up to 80 percent of mothers; if you experience the blues, you are not alone. Keep in mind these mild symptoms last only a week or two and go away on their own.[37]

Postpartum Depression Symptoms

Postpartum depression may be mistaken for baby blues at first. But the signs and symptoms are more intense, last longer, and, eventually, interfere with your ability to care for your baby and handle other daily tasks. Symptoms usually develop within the first few weeks after giving birth but may begin later—up to six months after birth.[38]

Symptoms may include:

- Depressed mood or severe mood swings
- Excessive crying
- Difficulty bonding with your baby
- Withdrawing from family and friends
- Loss of appetite or eating much more than usual
- Inability to sleep (insomnia) or sleeping too much
- Overwhelming fatigue or loss of energy
- Reduced interest and pleasure in activities you used to enjoy
- Intense irritability and anger
- Fear that you're not a good mother
- Feelings of worthlessness, shame, guilt, or inadequacy
- Diminished ability to think clearly, concentrate, or make decisions
- Severe anxiety and panic attacks
- Thoughts of harming yourself or your baby
- Recurrent thoughts of death or suicide

Untreated, postpartum depression may last for many months or longer.[39]

The very damaging, frightening part of postpartum is the lack of perspective and the lack of priority and understanding what is really important. —Brooke Shields

The feelings of sadness and anxiety with postpartum depression can be extreme and usually require treatment. Be sure to talk about how you are feeling with your doctor.

Postpartum Anxiety (PPA)

While postpartum depression and the so-called baby blues are widely discussed, postpartum anxiety, which many moms experience, is not as well known. We are aware of the warning signs for postpartum depression—such as prolonged sadness and excessive crying. But anxiety combined with PPD is even tougher to handle.

Postpartum anxiety affects about 10 percent of postpartum women, who may experience anxiety by itself or along with depression.[40] Postpartum anxiety can also include postpartum panic disorder, which includes having panic attacks along with feelings of anxiety.

Signs and symptoms may include:
- Eating and sleeping changes
- Feeling constantly worried
- Having racing thoughts that are tough to control
- Feeling scared that something bad will happen
- Tough time sitting still
- Dizziness, hot flashes, and nausea[41]

Postpartum Psychosis

With postpartum psychosis—a rare condition that typically develops within the first week after delivery—the signs and symptoms are even more severe.

Signs and symptoms may include:
- Confusion and disorientation
- Obsessive thoughts about your baby
- Hallucinations and delusions
- Sleep disturbances
- Paranoia
- Attempts to harm yourself or your baby[42]

Postpartum psychosis may lead to life-threatening thoughts or behaviors and requires immediate medical treatment.

When to See a Doctor

There is no simple test for a diagnosis of depression. Doctors look for a number of the common symptoms listed above. If you experience the symptoms of postpartum depression listed above for more than two weeks, talk to your doctor. If you have symptoms that suggest you may have postpartum psychosis, again, get help immediately.

It's important to call your doctor as soon as possible if the signs and symptoms of your depression have any of these features:
- Don't fade after two weeks
- Are getting worse
- Make it hard for you to care for your baby
- Make it hard to complete everyday tasks
- Include thoughts of harming yourself or your baby
- Are accompanied by suicidal thoughts

If ever you have thoughts of harming yourself or your baby, seek help *immediately*. Call your partner or a family member or friend to help you with your baby while you take care of yourself. Call your doctor, a health care provider, or even an emergency number like 911 or a suicide hotline number.

People with depression may not even realize or recognize that they're depressed. If you are concerned that a friend or loved one has postpartum depression or is developing postpartum psychosis, help them seek medical attention right away.

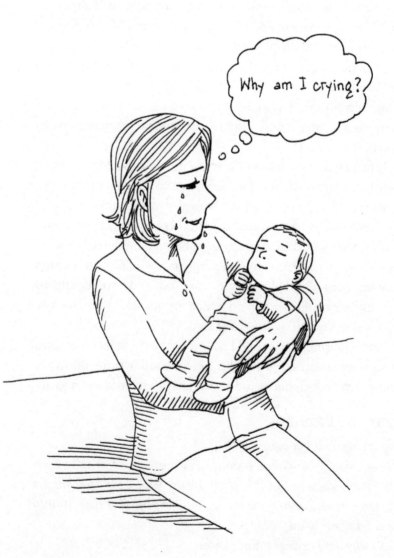

Stop Crying

I had mild anxiety along with postpartum depression. PPD and PPA can hit in varying degrees, but luckily for me, it was mild to moderate. In my case, the huge change was too much to handle. I was often alone with my own thoughts and rarely had any inter-action with people outside my immediate family. The feelings of isolation were overwhelming at times.

I worried about everything, from sleep to SIDS to breastfeed-ing. I worried about my baby's health and whether or not I was doing things right. I stressed about keeping the house in order, dropping the pregnancy weight, and looking attractive to my husband.

When I look back on those first few months, it saddens me that postpartum depression and anxiety took away some of the joys I would have liked to feel. I have struggled with depression since my twenties and have treated it with therapy and medication. I stopped taking medication before conceiving and hoped that the natural happy hormones during pregnancy would continue after baby was born. But that wasn't the case. I should have recognized the symptoms immediately and visited my doctor at the first signs; previous depression increases the risk of PPD.

I am a journal keeper, and I believe that writing is therapeutic. Though some entries during this time are sad, writing down my feelings gave me an outlet and a way to try to understand myself.

Journal Excerpt

Stop crying, I said to myself.

You should be happy, ecstatic. You are blessed. You've been given the miracle of life. A beautiful baby with ten perfect fingers and ten perfect toes and the most adorable little face that fits into the palm of my hand.

So why am I crying? I don't know!

The breastfeeding is exhausting me. My body feels depleted. As soon as I feed him, burp him, change him, and put him down to sleep, he's awake again.

I'm completely and utterly exhausted. I don't know if I can handle this.

Will I be a good mother? Will I be able to give him the best in life? This is the most important job in my entire life. I can't screw it up.

I just want to weep.

I have my mood swings like everyone else, and I'm having a moment.

I need to cry.

Let out some pent-up anger, frustration, bottled-up emotions.

Being strong is hard.

Crying is easy.

When I had these thoughts, I didn't want to hear about how grateful I should be. I didn't want to hear that tomorrow was another day or that I should stay positive. I just wanted to allow the tears to flow out of me and cleanse my spirit.

The sadness that I felt was overwhelming—not for any particular reason. It seemed to be an accumulation of realities, emotions, hardships, frustrations, disappointments, fears, and insecurities—one thing piled on top of another on top of another on top of another. I felt it was bound to fall and crash at some point. Putting on a facade of a superwoman could only last so long.

I felt like I was in a haze all the time, my brain foggy. I was in my own little world . . . just me and my baby in our safe cocoon, away from the real world. Other than caring for my baby and putting his needs first, I didn't care for much else. I felt exhausted due to lack of sleep and breastfeeding on demand and had little energy for anything else.

Mothers really were not built to raise babies not only by themselves, but with only a partner. For millions of years, a woman had much more than just her husband to help rear her young. . . . This whole idea of "It takes a village to raise a child" is exactly how we're supposed to live. —Helen Fisher

When you study postpartum depression, there is a very clear understanding that in communities where you see more support, there is less depression. —Ariel Gore

What Depression Feels Like

Depression is a dark and lonely place, like a dark cloud constantly hanging over your head. It truly does feel like you're trapped in a dark hole and you can't see the light. You start to look at people and the world as hopeless and see only the pain and suffering. You question life and what the whole point of it is. You feel utter dread.

When you're depressed, you no longer enjoy the simple things you used to look forward to: a morning cup of coffee, listening to music, cooking. Simple tasks like making the bed or putting together a nice outfit or a simple dinner can seem like a huge chore. You would rather sleep the day away—what's the point of getting up? For whatever reason—cultural, societal, self-inflicted pressures—new moms often feel a need to live up to a pedestal, to be a perfect mother and perfect wife who can do it all and do it all *well*. When these pressures build up, and you feel you are not *doing it all*, this contributes to PPD.

When I had my first son, there were no online support groups. I also was new to my area and hadn't made friends yet. My old friends didn't come around as much, and I felt they stayed away to give me space, but what I really needed was their company. Some friends who didn't have kids shied away . . . maybe they felt like they didn't know what to do or say or felt that staying away was what I wanted.

The truth is, I didn't know what I wanted at times. While I felt I needed to be alone, what I really needed was support. My feelings of loneliness even seemed confused, because when I did have visitors, I felt that was a burden as well.

In hindsight, I realize now that what would've made all the difference was practical support—family and friends who could come over and help me manage my home—fold laundry, cook dinner, and run errands while I rested, recovered, and took care of my baby.

My son was also colicky. That added to a very difficult first few months. Dealing with two to three hours of screaming a day took a toll very quickly. I questioned myself: *Am I doing something wrong? Why can I not comfort and soothe my baby?* These kinds of feelings can lead to worries that people think you're not doing a good job. If you have a postpartum disorder, you may struggle because you know you shouldn't care what people think but, ultimately, you fear people are judging you. You feel pressure to show the world that you have it all together, when in truth you doubt your ability to be that perfect mom the media portrays.

You may feel anxiety when you leave the house for simple errands. For me, the anxiety rushing through my body when I had to go out with the baby was insurmountable. I worried: *What if I have to change his diaper and there is no changing table? What if I struggle to open or close the stroller? What if he starts crying in the store? What if I have trouble getting him to breastfeed in public? What if he starts to wail in the car seat?*

The hassle just to get prepared to go out of the house took longer than the outing itself. With all the anxiety of taking baby out, I preferred to stay home. I isolated myself even more, which impacted my feelings of depression. It was a difficult cycle. I needed help.

When I finally went to see my doctor and she asked "How are you really feeling?" I burst into tears. I didn't have a clear answer as to why I was crying. According to people around me, I had no reason to be feeling depressed—I felt a deep sense of sorrow, but there wasn't a clear, defining reason. The melancholy had taken over, and I couldn't simply shake it off.

That's the thing with depression—you can't just wake up and decide not to be depressed. You can't just will yourself to be more positive. The brain is such a complex organ. Some fail to realize that mental illness, just like a physical illness, is real. There is no shame in getting help.

When I was contemplating antidepressants, I remember my doctor making the decision so simple; she said, "People take medication for their heart condition, or diabetes—so why would you question taking it for your brain?"

Finally, I went on medication, and it was as if the thunderstorm had ended and the sun started to shine through the clouds. The fog that occupied my head for months finally cleared. I felt normal again—not happy, because the medication just takes the edge off—but my normal self.

You are not alone.

To Moms

Dear New Mommy,
   Congratulations on your new bundle of joy. The moment you've been anticipating for more than nine months of

cravings, nausea, stretch marks, cankles, ultrasounds, listening to heartbeats, feeling baby kicks, nursery preparations, breathing, and a rollercoaster of emotions has finally arrived . . . now what?

It's just the blues, you tell yourself, crying and laughing within the same breath. It'll pass, they say, and for most new moms, it does after a short time. But you can't shake it. It's not getting better. Weeks have passed and you should be happy—you have a beautiful baby—but you're just not. Your baby is perfect, but you're not perfectly fine.

Postpartum depression is a beast. It will rob the moments that are supposed to be joyful with your baby. Don't wait to see your doctor. Get help right away. When you are well mentally and emotionally, you can enjoy your baby as you're meant to. Go see your doctor; you may need medication to help you through this time. It is okay to take medicine for a headache. It is okay to take medicine for PPD.

Gather your support team. There are people who would love to help you but likely don't know you are struggling. Talk to your spouse and let him know your needs and concerns. Join with a support group if there is one in your area. Look to family and friends for help too. You'll probably find that some struggled with the blues or PPD and know just how to help you get through it.

If you feel exhausted and cranky due to the lack of sleep and maybe lack of wholesome food, too, and maybe because you're a new mom and it's just hard, ask for help—even an hour—so you can take a nap, get a shower, and have a bite to eat.

You're meant to enjoy the newborn smell, the cuddles and coos. Even when you will feel that immense need to take a break, it's okay. You're still a good mother.

When you come out of the big blur, when you get some more sleep, when you get the hang of the diapering, feeding,

burping, swaddling routine, you will come out of that zombie-like slumber.

In time, you will feel as if you're coming back into your
own body and mind again.

You will come out of the darkness and enjoy the light
again—I promise.

—From one mama to another.

Chapter Ten

TAKING CARE OF MOM
IS IMPORTANT, TOO

Being a mother is hard, constant work. It's easy to fall into the habit of not caring for yourself as you put your baby's needs first. Most of your focus will be on caring for your child. But a mom who is well rested, enjoys a healthy diet, exercises, has social interactions with friends, and asks for help when she needs it is far more equipped to be the best mom she can be than a mom who puts her needs last.

How to do this? First, you need to manage expectations—your own as well as those thrust on you by others. Second, realize the importance of taking time for self-care and do NOT feel guilty about it.

Managing Expectations

Before I became pregnant, I had a notion that I was *supposed* to be a natural mom—I expected to morph into a supermom overnight. I imagined that I'd be able to do it all and handle it all: motherhood, career, and home life. When I actually became a mother, I started to think about why I had these preconceived ideas about being able to handle all of the responsibilities and challenges with ease. Did I put the pressure on myself? Did I perceive pressure from my husband and family? The media? I'm not looking to put the blame on anyone or point fingers, but you have to wonder where all of these expectations—unrealistic expectations—originated.

Media's depiction of motherhood is deceiving. You get only a partial picture—and it's usually a perfect one—of the woman who is juggling everything effortlessly. When I was pregnant, I remember paying closer attention to images of confident super-moms in print ads, TV commercials, and magazines. I know for a fact they didn't do anything to boost my confidence in being a first-time mom or empower me. I'm pretty sure they were some-what responsible for the added pressure I felt.

Baby Dove in the U.K. conducted the "Perfect Mum" exper-iment in response to nationwide research of 3,000 first-time British moms. Nearly nine out of ten (88 percent) first-time moms feel pressure to be perfect. What do they say contributes to the pressure? Media representations of motherhood in magazines and newspapers (47 percent), images on social media sites like Instagram and Facebook (33 percent), and celebrity moms (28 percent) are the main factors.[43]

I think many women have the vision of having a wonderful birthing experience, a hands-on husband, and a supporting fam-ily. Some women expect to suddenly evolve into the motherhood role without a hitch, breastfeed naturally, and spend much of the day cuddling and playing with baby. It's disappointing then to have your plans go awry; the natural childbirth you hoped for ended up being a C-section, breastfeeding caused cracked and bleeding nipples, and the husband who was supposed to help you breathe through labor ended up passing out on the hospital floor. Guess what—this is the real normal.

While some cultures have become more modern, others are still very much entrenched in tradition. In my husband's and my own culture, women are still regarded as responsible for taking care of household chores and children. The house should be immaculate. If your house isn't sparkling clean, then you aren't a good mother. A good mother wouldn't have dirty floors and a dirty house, no . . . what a disgrace! A mother who would go out with her girlfriends instead of staying home with the kids? Terrible!

To top it off, women are expected to *naturally* move into the role of the perfect mother who can cook, clean, and take care of baby—and husband too. Motherhood *should* be second nature; women are multitaskers and can do it all. I'd hear other older ladies say, "She can handle it." I was a supermom before I even became a mom.

Moms Work More

While I came to terms with my new responsibilities and concerns as a mom, I began to realize that being a mom is an underappreciated "job." Your role as a mother and the work involved never ends; you can't clock out at five o'clock in the afternoon. You care for your baby all day and night, and there are few breaks in between where you can actually relax. You can never let your guard down even for one second.

When someone asks "What did you do all day?" you want to punch them in the face and say, "I changed a gazillion diapers, fed my baby, whom I held in my arms for most of the day, and scrubbed spit-up off my shirt"—but it doesn't quite sum it up!

Depleted Mom Syndrome

As moms, we're typically conditioned to put ourselves last. We take care of ourselves once everyone else is taken care of. But by the time everyone else is taken care of, there is little time, motivation, or energy left to care for ourselves. Many moms today are running on empty and feeling overwhelmed and exhausted as they strive to do it all. Over time, those feelings of unhappiness and lack of fulfillment creep up, because we've neglected ourselves for too long. We are not eating well, not getting any exercise or sleep, and feel overwhelmed and overscheduled. We are left depleted.

If we don't take care of ourselves, how will we be healthy and well enough to care for our family? The problem with doing it all and doing it perfectly is that the high demand becomes stressful physically, mentally, and emotionally. Over time, your body and mind begin to break down—you can't keep up with the stress and pressure. You'll simply burn out.

In addition, stress, which is a natural side effect of being overwhelmed, affects the immune system, lowering our resistance to illness and disease. It also affects our sleep, diet, energy, hormones, menstrual cycles, and even libido. Stress has such a negative impact on so many aspects of our physical body and mental well-being.

As women, we have to empower ourselves to overcome the 24/7 demands and expectations that prevent us from being the moms we want to be. We need to adjust our expectations and see that the most important things—Mom and baby—are cared for first.

Ask yourself these questions:

- Why have you put such high expectations on yourself?
- Are your current goals realistic?
- Do you feel inadequate if you don't complete your list?
- What can you let go of to have more time to focus on those things that really matter?

- Are you concerned about what other people say?
- Are you afraid to say "no"?
- Are you ready to change your outlook, goals, and expectations for the sake of your health and well-being?

Rick Hanson, PhD, a psychologist and author, and his wife, Jan Hanson, an acupuncturist and nutritionist, have written and lectured extensively on parental stress and depletion, ways to nurture mothers and fathers, and how a husband and wife can be both strong teammates and intimate friends while raising a family. Their book *Mother Nurture: A Mother's Guide to Health in Body, Mind, and Intimate Relationships* introduces the term "depleted mom syndrome"—also known as "supermom syndrome" or "martyr syndrome."

The causes—physical, psychological, and social—include lack of sleep and exercise, poor diet, hormonal imbalances, nutrient loss, neurotransmitter deficiencies, guilt, anxiety, conflicting role expectations, marital conflict, and a breakdown of social supports. Symptoms include chronic fatigue, susceptibility to illness, connective tissue problems—including back pain and headaches—emotional numbing, depression, mood swings, irritability, hopelessness, confusion, running battles with husbands, and turning inward and away from friends and family.[44]

Basic baby care takes a lot of energy. Breastfeeding takes a quarter of your total caloric intake, which means many nutrients are depleted. Hormones impact brain chemistry and affect mood, sleep, and depression, which all play a factor in depleted mom syndrome. Baby at six months is still waking up to feed at night; lack of sleep can make anyone irritable, cranky, and short tempered. So when your fuse is blown, you end up snapping at your husband. There is an overall feeling of stress to accomplish the housework, make dinner, take care of demanding baby, and also perform in the bedroom.

Depleted mom syndrome is real! If you are concerned that you aren't handling motherhood as well as you expected, I hope you'll take comfort in knowing that you're not alone.

I Burned Myself Out

When I had my first child, I took the role of motherhood *extremely* seriously. I felt that it was my choice to bring a baby into this world, so I had a major responsibility to be the most prepared and educated parent. In my eyes, raising a child—to nurture, guide, provide, and love—is the greatest honor of my life. So in my first year of being a mother, I didn't go anywhere without my baby. I felt I had to be there for him every minute of the day. Call it territorial like a mama bear, but I felt like it was my responsibility. I had a tough time saying "yes" when family would offer to watch the baby. I thought: *I should be able to do this all on my own! Isn't that my job now? I'm the mother. I'm supposed to be with my baby 24/7.* If I would have left him in someone else's care, I would worry: *What if he's hungry? He wouldn't take to the bottle. What if my mom or husband can't get him to calm down?* While these are normal things to worry about, I allowed these worries to make time off for me impossible.

I put pressure on myself to be some kind of superwoman and supermom. In truth, I put the pressure on myself. I caved into cultural and media expectations.

In addition, breastfeeding left me exhausted. I wasn't eating properly, and my hormones were out of whack. I wasn't getting enough sleep. And I was suffering postpartum depression. I entertained too much when I should have said "NO." I didn't accept help when it was offered. I wanted people to think that I could handle it.

I felt like I was battling the challenges on my own. My husband was busy working to provide financially for the family, so some parenting decisions were left to me. *Do I try the Ferber method? Am I doing the right thing by trying attachment parenting?*

Although I realized I NEEDED a break, I felt extreme guilt that I was desperately seeking some time for myself. Then I hit a brick wall. I burned myself out. I literally felt like I had snapped—something in my mind switched. I can actually remember when and where it just seemed to suddenly click. It was a blustery winter day, and I was sitting at my desk in my office, staring out the window in a complete haze. I felt I knew I had to make a change or I wouldn't survive. And so I did.

When my second son turned one, I stopped breastfeeding after getting hit with mastitis several times (which knocked me off my feet). That was the pivotal point. Shortly after, I started a blog as an outlet to share my own motherhood/parenting stories in hopes that other women would realize they weren't alone. I joined the gym, putting my sons in daycare so I could exercise—I had to prioritize physical and mental health. And I lost the pregnancy weight. Once I was able to get my health in check, I feel like I found myself again.

Mom Guilt

If you've never experienced feelings of guilt before becoming a mother, you will soon learn what guilt feels like! It's probably one of the crummiest feelings you could inflict on yourself.

If you allow yourself to feel soul-crushing guilt for every choice you make as a parent, it will take a toll. Whether you're not able to calm your baby down or you've had to stop breastfeeding, there will be a myriad of reasons you may feel inadequate and guilty.

I'd have to say the one thing that causes women the most guilt is returning to work. Making the decision to pass your child over into the care of another person is the toughest, most heartbreaking choice to make as a woman. Your instincts are screaming at you to stay with your child, but financially you know you have to provide for that child. Working moms feel incredible guilt for needing or wanting to work. Women may have the desire to further their careers at a job they love while taking care of their family. Mom will feel guilty for leaving her child at daycare and then feel guilty for loving her job.

We have to stop thinking that to be a good mom, you must sacrifice everything you desire in order to take care of your children. This way of thinking is not only self-damaging but also detrimental to your child in the long term. You need to enjoy a meaningful, fulfilling life as well. Yes, we are responsible for caring for our children's needs. We also have a responsibility to care for ourselves as well.

Women also experience feelings of guilt when comparing themselves to other women and their parenting styles. "Oh look, she gets to breastfeed, but I can't" or "She gets to stay home and do crafts with her kids while I go to work." It's easy to come to conclusions about someone else's life based on your own perception (or that staged photo in a magazine), but it may not be the truth. The grass isn't always greener. Try to focus on what works for you and your family.

Burn the Supermom Cape

Ladies, it's time to throw away the supermom cape.

You may have to change your mindset and start being more realistic. You will not have the same time or energy to do the things you used to do before baby arrived. It is not humanly possible to do everything all at once.

In order to be in optimal health and take care of yourself, you will need to let some things go. What can you let go of? If finances are an issue, make a list of things you can cut down on in your budget in order to find extra income to pay for needed help. For

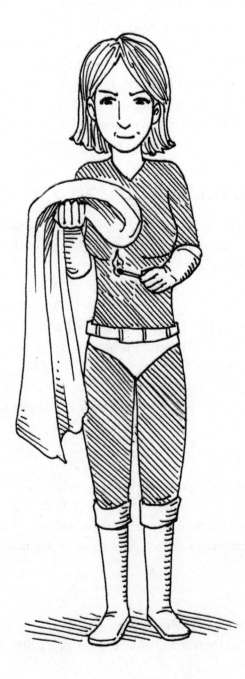

example, ditch the takeout dinners and use that money instead for a laundry service or meal-delivery service.

If keeping the home tidy proves to be a challenge, consider hiring a cleaning lady or a part-time mother's helper so you can get your errands done. It may be helpful to give up the Starbucks coffees—that's five dollars a day—and put that money toward a babysitter. Figure out what you need *most*, and go from there.

Let's start with some musts for taking care of Mom.

11 Tips on Taking Care of YOU

If only I had this list when I had my first child, maybe it would have helped me to put myself on the top of the scale *beside* my baby, not at the bottom.

Get More Sleep.

Take a nap when your baby/toddler naps. Who cares if housework is piling up? You need this rest. The more sleep you get, the more you can function normally . . . without wanting to tear off your husband's head. If you've had a nap—even just a twenty-minute power nap—you will feel more energized to conquer the rest of your household tasks.

Eat Well.

Eat a balanced, healthy diet and take a multivitamin. I can't stress enough how important it is to find the time to sit down and have a proper, nutritious meal. Especially if you are breastfeeding, you need those extra calories to help with milk production and to refuel.

Exercise.

Although it's difficult enough to find any free time, keeping your body healthy and active will also help you feel better and boost your energy. If you can't join a gym, get together with other moms for simple exercises like stroller walking. Physical activity also helps keeps your mental health in check. Just thirty minutes of walking, biking, or Pilates will improve your outlook.

Meditate.

Take up yoga, meditation, or any other form of a stress reliever. Ten minutes of quiet and deep breathing will help clear your mind and relax your spirit.

De-stress.

Even fifteen minutes a day—a bubble bath or reading a book—can help you unwind and de-stress. Research shows that just a five-minute walk in nature helps mental health.[45] Whether you head to the woods or a field, the beach, or the local park, your spirits will be lifted. Scientists tell us it works!

Just say NO!

You will be pulled in a hundred different directions and invited to family functions and friends' events. You will want to entertain but feel too tired. Although your heart is in the right place, you just can't do it all. Learn to say "no" to commitments. Don't try to do everything, or you'll end up feeling stressed out.

Simplify Household Chores.

Find products/ways to help do the job faster and easier. Schedule cleaning tasks to a specific day of the week to help keep you organized. Make a to-do list for your husband to tackle on the weekend. If financially possible, hire someone to clean the house every two weeks. There are great web sites like flylady.com or apps like the Cozi Family Organizer that can help with organization and quick cleaning. Just be careful not to feel like you need to do everything those websites suggest.

Ask for Help.

Don't be afraid to ask for help. Call your mom or mother-in-law to give you a hand. Family far away? Find a local babysitter or a high-school student helper. Or if you have a group of mom friends with young ones, take turns watching the kids so each of you can have an hour or two to run errands or simply take a nap. Don't overlook your partner as a great helper to watch baby while you get out for a bit. Some women fear that their hubby will struggle with a diaper change or not know what to do if baby is crying, but men are quite capable, and doing a little coaching can yield great rewards for Mom—and Dad, too!

Socialize.

Just because you've had a baby doesn't mean you can't still have a social life. Join a women's book club, visit a mom-and-baby group, or go out for a girls' night out—you need it!

Have Date Nights.

You'll also need to spend some time alone with your husband. Once the baby arrives, it's all about the baby . . . some couples tend to lose a little bit of their relationship and need to remember their relationship deserves attention too. A date night every so often can help rekindle the romance you had before the baby arrived.

Get Support.

Support can come from friends, parents, a counselor, or support groups, both in person and online. Meet other moms in your area and participate in open discussions—you'll be surprised how many moms feel exactly as you do!

Finding time for yourself when you're a new mom can seem nearly impossible. But if you want to take care of your family well, you'll quickly come to the realization that you must take care of yourself too! Mom's self-care shouldn't lead to feelings of mom guilt either; know that taking that time to feel your best is crucial so that you can be the best mom for your baby.

Mom to Mom

I would watch Gilmore Girls *(the original show) every afternoon while my baby girl was napping in her swing chair. It was the best therapy for me!* —Delia Rusu

If somebody offered to watch my son and let me go take a nap or a shower, I asked them if they were serious and then took them up on it. I learned to accept the help I was offered instead of always trying to do it myself, and by doing that, I allowed myself half an hour to an hour here and there to sneak in a little time for me where I could (in between nursing sessions). —Monica Bertenshaw

Take a long bath or shower or go for a walk solo—that's about all you get time for! —Nikki Stefancic

My friend Brenda and I used to meet at each other's houses with our wee babes. I would leave my kiddo with Brenda while I went out and ran for thirty minutes. Then I could take a quick shower. In that time, Brenda would be watching the kids. Then it would be Brenda's turn. When the kids were old enough for jogging strollers, we could go together, but each would watch the other's kid while the other had a shower. The alternative to this was that one of us could run errands in the thirty-minute run time . . . or nap. —Shannon Harris

Chapter Eleven

HOW TO SOOTHE BABY . . . AND YOURSELF, TOO!

I don't know why they say "you have a baby." The baby has you.

—Leo Gallagher

She has you—she sure does.

One of the toughest parts of parenting is dealing with a crying baby, especially when you can't figure out how to soothe him. Like every parent, you will become overwhelmed and even frustrated when your baby is crying.

Women naturally respond to baby's cries with sympathy and caring. A study showed that women who listened to the sounds of a baby crying in hunger showed a change in activity in certain brain regions, but men showed no change. Women are hardwired to respond strongly to the sound of baby's cries, making us more attentive and priming our bodies to help.[46]

Naturally, we rush to baby to try and soothe him. The stress associated with baby's cries can eventually take a mental and emotional toll; mom will have moments of needing some soothing too. You feel helpless because you want to comfort them but you're not sure how. Then you start to question your role as a mother and whether you're cut out for this entire parenting gig.

You'll soon come to realize that your baby will cry for a variety of reasons—not because they're sad or distressed (like adults). Babies will cry when they're tired, wet, hungry, or overstimulated. Think of crying as a way of baby trying to talk to you. Your baby will cry in order to communicate since she can't do anything for herself and will be relying on you to provide her with comfort, warmth, and, of course, nourishment. Crying is your baby's natural way of communicating her needs, so Mom and Dad will have to listen for cues and respond accordingly.

Did baby have an explosion in his diaper? Is he wet? But I just fed him! Why won't he stop crying? There were times I was at my wit's end trying to get my baby to calm down. The screaming cries that would pierce my eardrums, poking my brain like a woodpecker on bark until I was reaching for the pain reliever . . . and those earplugs.

Did I say it would be easy figuring out what your baby is trying to tell you? The truth is, it will be difficult at first. But when your sanity depends on helping baby feel peace—so you can too—you will figure out baby's crying language. Soon enough, you will recognize what your baby needs by the sound of her cries. Her cry may sound like a whimper when she wants to be held or a horror-movie-inspiring shrill when she's suddenly hungry for milk. You'll come to realize what your baby needs, and, as she grows, she'll learn other ways of communicating with you. Knowing the cues will help you realize how to respond and reduce your stress level.

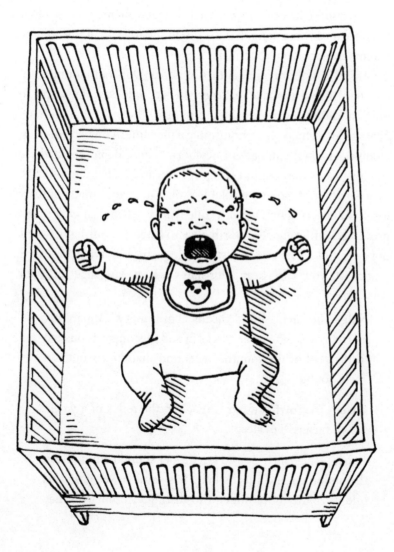

Five Types of Newborn Cries

When the Boss was four months old, we joined a Mother Goose program hosted at the local library with about eight other moms and babies. When one baby started to fuss and cry, the others would then join in! It was the funniest thing to hear a symphony of baby cries with different tones—some cries were high, others low. I would've loved to record each one and then edit it together to create a baby cry song. (Add a rap to the track, and it would be a number one hit on YouTube!)

Australian mom and author Pricilla Dunstan, founder of Dunstan Baby Language, believes she has unlocked the secret to understanding newborn babies' cries. Her theory is that all newborns from birth to three months have the same five newborn cries, a universal secret language of newborn babies. Babies make these sounds just as they begin crying. If you can satisfy them quickly, they won't erupt into inconsolable wails. Dunstan gained popularity after appearing on *Oprah*. While Dunstan Baby Language isn't proven scientifically, it is worth a try to listen to your baby's various cries and see if you can distinguish the meanings among them.

See if you can hear Dunstan's secret language in your baby's cries:

Neh—The "neh" sound means "I'm hungry." Apparently as a baby's sucking reflex kicks in and the tongue is pushed to the roof of the mouth, the sound that comes out is a "neh" sound.

Owh—The "owh" sound is made in the reflex of a yawn, which means "I'm sleepy."

Eairh—The "eairh" sound is a deeper sound coming from the abdomen and means baby has some lower gas. This one is a little more difficult to distinguish, but you may notice baby is pulling knees up or pushing legs down, and baby's face will look uncomfortable too.

Eh—The "eh" sound means that a baby needs to burp. When you hear "Eh, ehhhhh" your newborn is telling you they need to be burped. It sounds close to "neh" and "heh," but keep a close ear to the beginning sound, not the ending sound.

Heh—The "heh" sound (similar to "neh," so be careful that you hear the beginning h sound) means discomfort. That h sound at the beginning suggests that baby is uncomfortable, whether he's cold or hot, in an uncomfortable position, or needs a diaper change.[47]

Why Is Your Baby Crying in the First Place?

Whether or not you can hear Dunstan's sounds, your baby's cries communicate to you their needs. She may be trying to say one of the following.

Give Me Milk

Hunger is one of the most common reasons that your newborn baby will cry. The younger your baby is, the more likely that she's hungry. You may as well just plop down on the couch and remain there for the first three months of her life, because you'll be constantly feeding, whether by breast or bottle.

So you may as well make the most out of being on the couch. Make sure to have a book, journal, laptop or tablet, earbuds, and TV remote nearby. Some ideas to keep your mind occupied:

- Read a good book. It's a great escape from the burping, feeding, and diaper changing.

- Listen to your favorite podcast.
- Watch a funny TV show or movie and laugh.
- Call your mom or a friend.
- Do a crossword puzzle.
- Listen to some music.
- Write in your journal.
- Waste some time on Facebook.
- Close your eyes and rest. You'll feel better for it.
- Meditate. Breathe deeply.
- Enjoy the snuggly time with baby.

I'm Sleepy

There's a reason why you see newborn babies depicted in movies as always sleeping, because the first few weeks of their lives, that's all they do! When my boys were newborns, they slept most of the time. Newborns will either be sleeping, eating, or pooping!

As they get older, though, babies can have some difficulty getting to sleep, especially if they are overtired. Are they fighting sleep? You'll feel frustrated and exhausted because you're doing everything you can to lull baby to sleep, but she just won't close her eyes.

What worked for me? Swaddling baby with his legs flexed worked for my eldest, but my youngest would always kick off the blankets! The cutest thing is to see a baby kicking their legs like they're on *Dancing with the Stars*, their chubby rolls jiggling with every kick. Since the swaddle didn't work with my second baby, I'd hold him on one side of my body with his side facing outward and swing him side to side or back and forth. At the same time, I'd make a very annoying yet effective shushing sound. I'm telling you, it works.

Harvey Karp, author of *The Happiest Baby on the Block*, says the best way to calm your newborn and get him to sleep is by recreating the noises, movement, and snug environment of the womb by saying "shhh" into your swaddled baby's ear as you hold her on her side or tummy.[48] Shush as loudly as your baby is crying; as she calms down, lower the volume of your shushing to match. I know; it can be super annoying, especially when you need to do this while you're at the grocery store. I'd suggest not worrying about what people think and doing what you have to do to calm baby down and keep your stress level under control. Even if people think you are weird, they will see that your technique brings great peace to all in the room. Way to go, Mom!

Once you become aware of your baby's cues, you'll know when she's ready for a nap. The first few months when friends and family are visiting nonstop, your baby can become overstimulated and need some quiet to settle down. When she starts to whimper, yawn, and stare blankly into space, you know it's time for sleep. Don't delay sleep, because when baby becomes overtired, it will take even longer to get her to settle down for a nap. Let your visitors know it's time for them to leave so baby—and Mommy—can take a nap. As soon as you see the first signs of tiredness, jump on it! Otherwise, you may have a cranky pants on your hands.

I Did a Poopy

Check your baby's diaper. Is it too wet? Fitted too tight? Does she have diaper rash? Sometimes even letting baby free without a diaper is a good idea. Just make sure you have a towel underneath her—she may decide to pee. When out at Grandma's or Auntie's house, use a hospital pad or pet pad (available at pharmacies and pet stores) under baby when she needs a little less restriction.

I'm Hot; I'm Cold

Some babies would rather not be naked. Your baby may not be a big fan of baths or having a diaper change. I wouldn't like to be sitting naked on a change table with my legs up and a cold wipe on my bare bum either! Make it quick. Have everything ready so you can get baby dressed quickly again.

I've found keeping the bathroom warm when you give baby a bath and wrapping her in a warm towel once you take her out of the water can help. You'll get used to bathing and changing your baby quickly with practice.

Pay attention to your baby's temperature. You can check how hot or cold the baby is by feeling her stomach—not her hands or feet, as they usually feel cool to the touch. If her tummy feels too hot, remove a layer, and if it feels cold, add a layer. Usually one more layer of clothing than you are comfortable wearing is just right for your baby.

During summer months, baby may need nothing more than a diaper—you can always try removing a layer to see if baby is more content. If you are hot and would remove another layer—if only it were not illegal—perhaps baby can just bare all. There are few times in life when this is acceptable, so let him take advantage.

I Don't Feel Well

If baby is under the weather, her cry might sound different too. The tone may be higher or lower pitched, stronger, or even weaker. If your baby cries a lot but suddenly is quiet, it could also mean she is not feeling well. Mama's instinct is so often right, so if you feel like something could be wrong, I'd suggest calling or going to visit your doctor.

When the Boss was four months old, the sound of his cry changed in volume, from head-exploding high to whimpering weak. I knew something was wrong and took him to the pediatrician. Soon enough, he developed a fever and rash. The illness turned out to be roseola, a virus that most commonly affects young children between six months and two years old. Roseola is usually marked by several days of high fever followed by a distinctive rash just as the fever breaks.

While Google can be your best friend, the information you find may not always be accurate and should never act as a substitute for a physician's diagnosis. The Boss technically was too young to have roseola according to the internet, and yet that is exactly what his illness turned out to be.

Babies often cry because they have an ear infection or cold or even have fallen and injured themselves (don't leave baby unattended on a bed). Visit the doctor if your baby is showing signs of illness or injury and your motherly instincts are nagging you.

C'mere and Cuddle with Me

Your baby will want and need a lot of cuddling. This is the fun part! The close physical contact is reassuring and comforting. Even adults love being held and cuddled. We need lovin' too! Baby will grow accustomed to the sound of your voice and your smell, especially the smell of breast milk. Baby will love to look at mom's or dad's face when being held.

Don't waste even a moment worrying whether you are spoiling your baby by holding her too much—that's a ridiculous myth. I remember hearing people tell me, "It's not good to always be holding the baby or letting the baby sleep on you." I'd roll my eyes at this incorrect advice.

Drs. William and Martha Sears, authors of *The Attachment Parenting Book*, say that attachment parenting implies responding appropriately to your baby; spoiling suggests responding inappropriately.[49] During the first several months of life, a baby's wants are a baby's needs, so responding to them with a "yes" teaches trust, which will make them more accepting of "no" later on. It's perfectly okay to say yes to baby's need to cuddle or be held close.

Cuddles also allow baby to feel soothed by the sound of your heartbeat. You can try holding her in a sling to keep her close to your chest. Babywearing is wonderful because baby can come on fun adventures with you: folding laundry, making the bed, and doing dishes—bubbles are the best! Teach him early on that household chores can be a riot! What's best, Dad can also hold baby close too. Babywearing provides a wonderful opportunity for Dad to bond and feel more involved with the baby.

*There isn't a more challenging sound for a new
parent than a baby screaming its lungs out for
three hours straight.*

I'm Weepy but I Don't Know Why

In the first three months, your baby may cry in the late afternoon and evenings *for no freaking reason*. It could range from short bursts of inconsolable crying to several hours at a time. Nothing can comfort him. You've tried changing him, feeding him, rocking him, and shushing him. Your baby may squirm, tighten his whole body by arching his back, draw his knees up to his chest, and clench his fists.

Wiki Fact

> *The word* colic *is derived from the ancient Greek word for
> "intestine" (sharing the same root as the word* colon*).*

Baby colic is defined as episodes of crying for more than three hours a day more than three days a week for three weeks in a row in an otherwise healthy child between the ages of two weeks and four months. It is present in 5 to 25 percent of infants.

My son was colicky and cried for about three hours every evening for the first three months. I was about to lose my mind. I would walk him up and down the hallway, holding him in every position imaginable, and when I was ready to throw in the towel, I handed him over to my husband. Once his shift was up, my mom took over. And so it went for weeks. *Weeks.* See your pediatrician to ensure there is nothing physically wrong with your baby. In fact, always check with your doctor if you aren't sure about your baby. While baby books and the internet may provide a wealth of knowledge and advice, it's always best to consult with your pediatrician.

With my firstborn, the pitch of his crying was fierce and high. It would start off low and then increase in volume and intensity. It's heartbreaking when nothing you do helps your baby stop crying.

If your baby can't settle down after being changed and fed, and even if your baby is colicky, the following calming measures may help.

Keep Moving

Try swaddling baby with the legs flexed and holding the baby on their side or stomach. Swinging the baby side to side or back and forth while supporting the head may help. Walking up and down the halls of the house or rocking your baby while making a shushing sound can also help. I've tried putting baby in a vibrating bouncy chair as well as a swing while supervising him. Some babies feel calm when they hear the hum or feel the vibration from the dryer or dishwasher.

Sometimes taking baby for a ride in the car can also help baby calm down. Take a drive in the country, stop for coffee along the way . . . maybe discover that new takeout dive off the highway and drive through for a bacon double cheeseburger with poutine!

Play Music

Music can help calm baby down. Is there a song you would listen to endlessly during pregnancy? It's known that babies can hear outside noises in the womb, although sounds are rather muffled. Try playing that sound or song again. According to research, when a baby hears music after the second half of pregnancy, any sound played frequently becomes learned.[50] So if baby hears the same sounds after birth, the baby seems to pay attention to it and quiet down.

Try some baby-friendly lullabies. But when the sing-along children CDs start burning a hole in your brain, switch to the radio. Introduce your little one to Metallica early on—whatever works to calm him.

One time when the Boss was crying uncontrollably, I turned on the stereo and scooped him up into my arms, and we danced around the family room. He immediately stopped wailing and stared at me like I had a second head growing out of my neck! His eyes opened wide, and then he finally started to smile. Finally, success! If music can lift me up and pull me out of a funk, it may help baby too.

Keep Her Sucking

Sometimes nursing baby skin against skin is soothing enough to help ease her cries. Multiple studies have shown that skin-to-skin contact between mom and baby during the first few weeks offers many benefits.[51] Even Daddy can participate by holding baby to his bare chest with baby wearing only a diaper; Dad will have to settle for offering a pacifier. But if it works and gives you a break, be sure to give Dad some awesomeness points.

In some newborns, the need to suck is very strong, and sucking can help baby settle down. While inside the womb, many babies suck their fingers or fists, as it steadies the heart rate and relaxes the body. Offer your breast, a pacifier, or a finger—but make sure it's scrubbed and washed clean first!

> *When your first baby drops her pacifier, you sterilize it. When your second baby drops her pacifier, you tell the dog: "Fetch!"—Bruce Lansky*

One time, an aunt of mine, God bless her soul, was holding my baby when he was just a few months old and she put her curled finger into his mouth. I was horrified! My neurotic first-time-mom personality lashed out, and I blurted, "Did you wash your hands?" I felt bad for being so bold, but I did not want to risk having germs passed on to my baby. My husband, who is even more neurotic than me, ensured that anyone coming in contact with our baby had washed their hands first before holding him.

Keep Calm

Take an infant massage class and learn how to massage your infant. Even gently rubbing her back or tummy might help. You can try playing white noise sounds, which mimic the sounds in the uterus. I'd suggest buying a CD with sounds of nature, downloading music of running water, or even meditation and yoga background music. Rather than "Mama" or "Dada," your baby's first word might turn out to be "Ooommm!"

You'll Need to Be Soothed, Too

You will also need to be soothed because you'll inevitably feel stressed. Remind yourself that you're not the reason your baby is crying and that the crying won't harm her in any way. You may have to accept that your baby is colicky or cries a lot and know that this phase will pass.

I spent a lot of time holding my baby, because every time I tried to put him down, he would start to cry. It wasn't until after the colic phase passed that baby enjoyed being in the bouncy chair or swing. Otherwise, it was mom and dad's arms only, and that became exhausting. There were many times I felt as if I was failing at motherhood; if I couldn't soothe my baby, then what did that say about my parenting skills?

You may find yourself sneaking to the bathroom to have a good cry because you're so frustrated! Releasing that pent-up sadness/irritation/negative energy can have amazing effects. You'll need to remind yourself that baby will cry, sometimes for no apparent reason. Still, you're a good mother! While you adore this little human with every fiber of your being, right now you need a time-out for yourself.

Place baby safely in her crib and give yourself a few minutes to de-stress. Go outside for a quick breath of fresh air or have a good cry. If possible, make a call and ask for help and support. A family member or a friend won't mind taking over for an hour while you take a break. Don't feel guilty about asking for help regularly—if you continue to let the stress build, you are doing yourself (and your baby) a huge disservice.

Caregivers, just like parents, can use some helpful tips on how to deal with a crying child. Taking care of a fussy baby or a baby who can't be consoled is very stressful. Make sure to communicate to your husband, family member, or babysitter what to do in the event that baby won't stop crying. Instruct them to put baby down in a safe place, take a break, and call you. Let them know to NEVER shake your baby. It takes only a few seconds of shaking to cause irreversible brain damage in an infant.

Mom to Mom

I asked a few moms what calmed their babies. Here are their replies:

When my baby was young (like zero to two months), John Denver music worked. It was super weird (because we never listen to John Denver normally), but whatever works!
—Jennifer Newberry

Self-soothing blankets and my hair kept my baby happy!
—Ashely Braun

I sing to them. I have three boys and would sing the alphabet in either French or English. Still works now too. They are eight, six, and two. —Jennifer Hunter-Pigeon

Being held close or carried in a front carrier worked for all of them. A warm shower with me holding him worked wonders for one. Simon & Garfunkel was a favorite as well!
—Denise Finlay Dodds

Breastfeeding was the only thing that ever made him happy! Could explain why he is still breastfeeding at almost twenty-eight months. —Rebeccah Beaulieu

When my daughter was really young, a pacifier and holding her and walking laps around the house soothed her. Now she's two and singing soothes her (no one else is allowed to hear it though!). —Lindsay Pevcevicius

Chapter Twelve

WHAT IS SLEEP?

*People who say they sleep like a
baby usually don't have one.*

Sleep was an issue for both of my children . . . in fact, I think it's more accurate to say it's an issue for most parents. For moms, the sleep issue begins before baby even arrives. During the second trimester, baby may begin to take up more room, resulting in nighttime visits to the bathroom. During the third trimester of pregnancy, Mom and Dad may as well say bye-bye to a good night's sleep for at least a year. *At least.*

Once baby comes around and takes over your entire life for those first few months, you will daydream about the days when you were a teenager and could sleep in until eleven o'clock in the morning. Those full eight hours of sleep that you so enjoyed and looked forward to on weekends? A distant memory. Now you're spending your life helping your baby fall asleep. And he will fight it, I'll tell you. The world is too exciting for sleep! There is too much to look at and explore! Since babies are stimulated constantly, it's no wonder they find it difficult to settle down. *Go to sleep, my baby, my baby, my baby. Just go to sleep! Please!*

After my children were born, I didn't sleep well for . . . I don't know; it's all a blur, really. "Sleeping in" meant I slept five hours straight *in my own bed*. While some may think five hours of total sleep is enough, when you're waking up two or three times within those five hours, it isn't very much at all. Lack of sleep means the likelihood of feeling irritable and cranky is sky high. The thought that it may be years before you have an opportunity to sleep in again is frightening!

Here's the good news: all babies eventually sleep through the night. Whether you wait for it to happen naturally or whether you wearily try different sleep techniques, it will happen. The first time baby sleeps a full five hours straight, you'll be running into his room wondering if he's still breathing. "Oh my gosh, is he alive?!" And you'll marvel when you realize that your baby is still asleep peacefully and you can enjoy a coffee all by yourself!

You'll update Facebook with the exciting status. *He did it! My baby slept five hours straight!* You'll feel refreshed and ready to conquer the day. With your newfound time and energy, you will be able to build a brand-new playground in the backyard and invent a new theory on time travel! Heck, you will even have time left over to write a chapter for your romance novel before baby wakes up!

But before you call the parade posse, know that tomorrow, he may just decide to wake up in the middle of the night again. And when baby is toddler age, he may still occasionally wake up. If you accept that there will be good days/nights and bad ones, you'll survive this parenting thing just fine.

There are hundreds of books published to help you help baby sleep. Authors and publishers know moms are desperate! Check out some of my favorite sleep classics.

Baby Sleep Books

- *Secrets of the Baby Whisperer: How to Calm, Connect, and Communicate with Your Baby* by Tracy Hogg and Melinda Blau
- *Solve Your Child's Sleep Problems* by Richard Ferber
- *Sleeping Through the Night, Revised Edition: How Infants, Toddlers, and Their Parents Can Get a Good Night's Sleep* by Jodi A. Mindell
- *The No-Cry Sleep Solution: Gentle Ways to Help Your Baby Sleep Through the Night* by Elizabeth Pantley
- *Healthy Sleep Habits, Happy Child: A Step-By-Step Program for a Good Night's Sleep* by Marc Weissbluth
- *The Sleepeasy Solution: The Exhausted Parent's Guide to Getting Your Child to Sleep from Birth to Age 5* by Jennifer Waldburger and Jill Spivack

How Much Sleep Babies Need

Birth to Three Months

Newborns sleep sixteen to seventeen total hours a day, but those hours of sleep are all broken up. Since newborns need to eat every two to four hours, most newborns sleep for only an hour or two at a time. Once your baby reaches about four to six weeks of age, they will sleep fourteen to sixteen hours a day. By eight weeks, some babies—not all—will start sleeping longer at night but will still wake up several times a night for feedings. It's too early to even consider beginning a sleep and feeding schedule, although it's acceptable to dream about sleeping through the night!

Since baby is sleeping and waking sporadically, it's important for mom to sleep as often as possible too. My suggestion? You'll be zombie-like for the first few months, so when your baby finally does settle down, take a nap with your baby—you'll feel refreshed and ready to continue with the rest of your day. The laundry can wait.

Three to Six Months

Around three or four months, the newborn phase is officially over! By now, your baby will likely begin a sleeping pattern of shorter daytime naps and longer periods of sleep at night. But be warned— not all babies are able to fall into a schedule of their own by this age. Be patient—that time will soon come.

While sleep at night will still include waking, naps may become more clearly defined. Babies at four months may have about four naps during the day; by six months, three or four short naps. Don't fret if the times of the naps vary day to day; some babies are predictable with naptimes, while others won't fall into a routine until later.

By about three to six months old, most babies will be sleeping through the night. Some babies won't—and that's perfectly okay . . . though likely not what you hoped for, it's completely normal. Your baby will likely be sleeping for longer periods through the night, so hopefully you're getting better stretches of sleep yourself and feeling better too!

Seven to Nine Months

By around seven months, most babies are having about two or three naps during the day, and by eight months, about two naps a day: a morning and afternoon nap. Just remember that all of a sudden, your baby may begin to wake during the night. This could be caused by teething or physical developments such as learning to crawl, stand up, cruise, and even take steps.

While one night feeding is still considered normal at this point, some experts recommend weaning the night feeding by nine months. Cutting out the night feeding will help you determine whether your baby is genuinely hungry or if your baby is waking more out of habit.

Ten to Twelve Months

By this age, most babies are sleeping through the night—hooray! Some babies will continue to need one night feeding up to twelve months. Most babies are taking two naps per day at ten months old. If your baby doesn't have a predictable daytime nap schedule, you can help to create one. This will help ensure that baby is sleeping enough during the day and at night.

Baby Sleep Chart

Age	Sleep (hours)	Naps (hours)	Total sleep (hours)
Newborn–2 months	8–9	7–9 (3–5 naps)	16–18
2–4 months	9–10	4–5 (3 naps)	14–16
4–6 months	10	4–5 (2–3 naps)	14–15
6–9 months	10–11	3–4 (2 naps)	14
9–12 months	10–12	2–3 (2 naps)	14

Sleep Deprivation

Everyone talks about how babies need better sleep, but what about parents? Of course new parents are sleep deprived—but do you know just how much?

According to a 2013 survey, new parents lose forty-four days in the first year of a newborn's life. New moms reported an average of five hours of sleep, three hours short of the recommended eight hours. That's a deficit of about twenty hours of sleep per week, about 1,055 hours, or forty-four days, in the first year of a newborn's life.[52] It's no wonder new parents are exhausted!

Breastfeeding moms suffer the most sleep loss, as newborns nurse every two to three hours, even at night. The National Sleep Foundation says that the average adult needs seven to nine hours of sleep per night.[53] When you're sleeping only a couple of hours at a time, "you build up a 'sleep debt' that can be hard to pay back."[54] Until baby is sleeping longer stretches during the night, and when you're sleeping less than what you need, you may be more irritable, short tempered, and vulnerable to stress. Here's the silver lining . . . around baby's half-year birthday, your dreams about sleeping longer will begin to come to fruition! As baby is sleeping longer stretches, so will you . . . and that milestone is something to celebrate.

Better Sleep for Mom

As you learn about baby's sleep, there are some tips that can apply to Mom's sleep too! Getting enough sleep is essential to your health and well-being and makes you a better parent.

Here are some ways to improve your sleep.

Have a Sleep Schedule

Go to sleep and get up at the same time every day.[55] Having a regular schedule helps your body's internal clock and improves how well you sleep. Choose a bedtime when you normally feel tired so that you're not lying awake for hours. If you're getting enough sleep, you should wake up naturally without an alarm. If you need an alarm clock, you may need an earlier bedtime.

Nap When Baby Naps

Nap when the baby naps, especially during the first three months when your baby is a newborn and waking up often to eat. If you can't fall asleep, at least rest—even if you're tempted to throw in a load of laundry or empty the dishwasher! I know; there will always be some household chore to catch up on. There will be some tasks you must complete while baby is sleeping, but one of your priorities should be to rest and sleep.

Although napping is a good way to make up for lost sleep, if you have trouble falling asleep or staying asleep at night, napping can make things worse. Power naps of fifteen minutes or so can do wonders, but longer naps can throw your sleep rhythms off.

Avoid Caffeine and Alcohol

Avoid caffeine, and that includes chocolate, tea, and soda, too! Caffeine does stick around in your bloodstream for a while, making it harder to sleep soundly. Also, alcohol may seem like it'll help make you feel drowsy, but more than a glass or two can have the opposite effect and disturb your sleep.

Exercise

Regular exercise can improve how well you sleep too. The key to using exercise to improve sleep is to maintain a regular pattern: thirty to forty-five minutes of moderate aerobic exercise three to five times a week. But don't work out too close to bedtime or else you'll feel too wired to fall asleep.

Create a Sleep-Enhancing Bedroom

Create a relaxing sleep environment. Is your mattress and pillow comfortable? Does your room have a window with blackout curtains? Your bedroom should be cool—between 60 and 67 degrees.[56] Consider using blackout curtains, eye shades, earplugs, white noise machines, humidifiers, fans, and other devices to help create a peaceful atmosphere that will help you sleep.

Establish a Bedtime Routine

While you're practicing a bedtime routine for your baby, you can do the same for yourself! Your own bedtime routine could include reading, listening to soft music, or having a warm bath or shower before bed.

These tips can help you to improve your own quality of sleep. Take the time for yourself, because a well-rested parent is also a happy one!

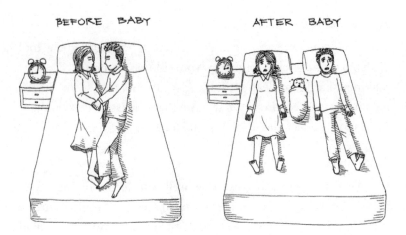

BEFORE BABY   AFTER BABY

Sleeping Through the Night

A question that many new parents hear often is "Does your baby sleep through the night?" Of course, the common answer is NO. Newborns wake up many times during the night to eat. Their small tummies aren't big enough hold large amounts of milk. Breast milk is digested quickly, so baby will breastfeed often—anywhere from every hour to every two to three hours. When you hear the term *sleep through the night*, this usually means a stretch of five hours— not the eight you were hoping for![57]

Most babies will wake up two to three times a night up to six months of age and once or twice a night up to one year old.

Set a Sleep Schedule

Sleep habits help parents as well as baby. When baby goes to bed before nine o'clock at night, babies tend to sleep better, according to research done by Dr. Jodi Mindell and others. In fact, according to the study entitled "Sleep and Social-Emotional Development in Infants and Toddlers" published in the *Journal of Clinical Child & Adolescent Psychology*, later bedtimes and less total sleep also causes children to feel separation distress, general anxiety, and depression/withdrawal.[58] Late sleepers may become overtired and find falling asleep difficult. While baby seems energetic late at night, it's often a sign that it's past her bedtime.

If parents use a consistent bedtime before nine o'clock at night—ideally between seven o'clock and eight thirty in the evening—babies will sleep better and longer.[59] This is great news for parents: putting baby to sleep sooner means he will sleep longer—and so will you!

Establishing a Bedtime Routine

You can begin a bedtime routine as early as you wish; however, any sleep-training method should not occur prior to six months.

Baby's bedtime routine can include a warm bath, changing into pajamas, reading a bedtime story (yes, even those first weeks—baby loves to hear your voice), singing a lullaby, giving baby a massage, and kisses and cuddles—in whatever order you wish. Keep the same routine each night and keep it under forty-five minutes. Whatever routine works for your family is fine, as long as you do it in the same order and at the same time every night. Even when your baby is unwell, do your best to maintain her usual routine. Here's an example of a bedtime routine that is simple and effective:

1. 7:15 p.m.: Feeding
2. 7:30 p.m.: Bath time, diaper, and pajamas

3. 8:00 p.m.: Bedtime story, cuddles, and kisses
4. 8:15 p.m.: Lay baby in crib; play music, rub her back

Naps

Set naptimes the same way you set bedtimes, but use a shorter nap routine. For example, keep the room quiet and read baby a story before patting baby on the back and leaving the room.

Plan naps for a specific time each day if you prefer a strict schedule, or follow your baby's cues—put her down when you know she's tired. You might notice she is closing her fists, yawning, fluttering eyelids, or seems to be staring into space.

I've heard stories of babies who refuse to nap more than a few minutes at a time but will sleep six hours straight during the night. Moms complain that they can't get anything done because their baby won't nap. Listen, ladies: you can't have it both ways! Be grateful that your baby is sleeping six hours straight at night! Find creative ways to get stuff done. Baby can hang out in his swing, in his bouncy chair, or even on his play mat while you zip around the house getting things done. At least you're not a zombie mom, walking around with bags under your eyes, bumping into furniture!

Other moms have babies who don't sleep well at night or for naptimes. It's just the way it goes. Be patient and try some different sleep-training techniques.

Trouble Sleeper

You know that moment when you put the baby down in his crib and slowly start tip-toeing away? Your toes touch the outside of the bedroom door and you think to yourself, *"Yeeeeeesssss, I'm free!"* It's as if baby knows you've crept away! Their little eyes flicker wide open, like one of those creepy old dolls from the 1970s. Then baby starts to wail.

Here are just a few of the common sleep problems parents of babies six months and older may face.

Baby Wants the Breast or Bottle to Fall Asleep

Change up the routine. If your baby is dependent on a bottle or breast to sleep, feed her before the bedtime routine. After cuddles and bedtime stories, place her in the crib, sleepy.

Babies will learn to soothe themselves. Of course, if your baby is used to feeding before bedtime, he will prefer a warm breast in his mouth while dozing off to dreamland. But many babies will learn to soothe by sucking on a thumb or a pacifier. Others may soothe to music, rocking themselves, or rubbing fingers on a soft blankie.

Once your baby learns to fall asleep on her own, you can go in at night if she wakes. Sleep experts will say you shouldn't pick her up or nurse her; your voice and a gentle stroke should be enough to get her settled into sleep once more.

Children who go to bed early get up early.
Children who go to bed late get up early. Um . . .

Baby Wakes Up Too Early

Early is a relative term. For some parents, a six a.m. wake-up time is ideal. But for others, any time before eight o'clock is considered too early. Is baby waking up after six o'clock happy, energized, and ready to go? Then you may not have an early rising problem! A wake-up time of six o'clock or later is reasonable for most babies provided they are getting enough sleep at night and during naptime.

If baby is waking earlier than six o'clock and doesn't last very long in the morning, and/or is cranky, then you may have an premature riser on your hands.

Experiment with an earlier bedtime. It may sound counteractive, but putting your baby to sleep earlier may mean longer and better sleep during the night. Try putting your baby to bed five minutes earlier every night until you reach the desired bedtime.

While every child is slightly different in terms of how much sleep they need, research shows that an early bedtime between seven o'clock and eight thirty works best for babies and kids through school age.

Baby Keeps Waking Up at Night

Make sure your baby's bedroom is dark at night, especially during summer. If baby wakes up early, offer a pat and a kiss and then leave the room. If baby starts crying, stay in the room but remain quiet, or "shush" baby back to sleep. You don't want to engage or excite baby; you're trying to affirm that it's still time for sleep.

When morning time does finally arrive, you can turn on the lights, open the curtains, and say a big "Good morning!" Doing these things consistently may help shift your child's morning wake-up time.

Street traffic, barking dogs, and chirping birds can wake a light sleeper from a deep slumber. Keep the windows closed, and try a white-noise machine or calming sounds throughout the night. Remind other children and your spouse to keep quiet as baby is sleeping. Dad: refrain from banging on the pots and pans, please! Leave a Post-it note on the stove and fridge as a reminder to use caution during early hours in the kitchen.

From the time my babies were newborns, I tried to keep the house volume as normal as possible so they'd become accustomed to the noises of regular household activity. But a telephone or doorbell ringing could easily wake them up from a deep sleep. Sometimes, a written note on the door saying "Please do not ring doorbell" and turning the telephone ringer to silent can help.

Is the Nap to Blame?

If your little one is sleeping too much during naptime, this may lead to too little sleep during the night. Try limiting naptime, but be careful—if your baby seems overtired by dinner time, he may still need a longer nap. When does baby's last nap end? Bedtime should begin about three to three-and-a-half hours after the last nap ends. If naptime doesn't begin until four thirty, it will be hard to get baby to bed on time.

The Boss was a serial catnapper. But the Underboss loved his afternoon nap. Still, when I started to make sure his afternoon nap began on time and limit the length of his nap, he started to sleep longer at night.

Nursing Time Is Not Sleep Time

If baby is falling asleep nursing and you let her sleep in your arms, she may be getting most of her sleep during those breastfeeding sessions. Help teach baby to sleep at nap and bedtime rather than eating time. Keep baby awake while nursing and then have some play time. Baby will nap and sleep better.

If All Else Fails . . .

The Boss wasn't the greatest sleeper, and sometimes his early waking and short daytime naps meant our days were pretty chill. Add the Underboss, my second boy, to the mix, and there were times when we all napped together for two hours in the afternoon. It worked for us, and was a phase when the phrase "this too shall pass" rang true.

My children's laughter is the best sound in the world.
The sound of them sleeping is second.

Sleep Training

Many parents struggle with a baby who either can't fall asleep on her own or wakes up frequently. Experts agree that the goal of sleep training is to help babies learn to self-soothe and fall asleep on their own at night.

There are several sleep-training methods out there—do your research, read about each method, and see what works for you.

Ferber Method

The popular Ferber method involves a bedtime routine of putting your child down at bedtime awake and checking on your child at set intervals (one minute, two minutes, three minutes, then every five minutes) until they fall asleep. When you check, the interaction should be very brief and without physical contact. The parent should say, "Goodnight. I love you. See you in the morning." This method is effective but can be challenging to carry out when baby cries.

After a few days to a week of gradually increasing the waiting time, most babies learn to fall asleep on their own, according to this theory. The baby realizes that crying means a parent will only check up on them, not pick them up.

The No-Cry Sleep Solution

The no-cry sleep solution is based on author and parent educator Elizabeth Pantley's set of techniques to change a baby's sleep habits without unnecessary tears. (Let's just say she's on the other end of the spectrum from Dr. Ferber when it comes to crying babes.) Pantley advocates a careful routine: pre-bedtime activities like bath, books, and lullabies to help a child prepare to fall asleep. Her book offers many tips to help babies (and parents) sleep with a *gentle* approach.

Pantley's book had a permanent home on the side table in the family room, and I lugged it with me upstairs to bed some nights.

I have highlighted excerpts in the book and tried every helpful tip. Persistence is key when it comes to sleep-training your child. I don't like the word "training" so much, as it's difficult to program a child to sleep and eat according to *your* schedule, because a baby's needs change over time.

Pantley offers a gentle and gradual approach to all aspects of sleep, customized to your baby's needs. She recommends rocking and feeding your baby to the point that he's drowsy before putting him down and responding immediately if he cries. Parents are urged to keep sleep logs, nap logs, and night-waking logs to document sleep patterns. She also suggests using "keywords" to signal to your child that it's time for sleep. While the gentle approach can take longer than the cry-it-out methods, no-tears advocates say it's less traumatic for baby and parents too! The best advice I can offer is to listen to your gut and do what feels right.

Dr. Jodi Mindell

Dr. Jodi Mindell, author of *Sleeping Through the Night: How Infants, Toddlers, and Their Parents Can Get a Good Night's Sleep*, offers four steps for helping establish baby's bedtime routine. Step one is to set a consistent bedtime every night to help set baby's internal clock. Step two is to establish a consistent bedtime routine. Step three is to establish a consistent bedroom environment, and step four is to put baby down awake so he can fall asleep on his own.[60] Dr. Mindell's method is gentle and simple, and many parents say it works!

Co-Sleeping

The truth about baby and sleep is, sometimes the techniques above don't work! Very few worked for my children. Both of my boys would scream their heads off when I put them down alone.

One night, my husband and I decided we would try the Ferber method. I had mentally prepared myself for the inevitable cries.

Though I hated the idea, I wanted to give it a whirl. Well, whadd'ya know—the Boss wailed for me to pick him up once he realized the lights were out and I was leaving the room. It sounded as if a bunch of raccoons were involved in a gang fight outside our window. I tried patting him on the back, shushing, playing music, speaking to him gently, etc., but his screams grew even louder. *Nope, can't do it! I'm so sorry, my baby!* I couldn't bear to hear his screams. I picked him up, took him to my bed, and that was the end of that. Trial concluded after ten minutes. Ferber just isn't well suited to some babies or parents.

My husband and I shared our bed with our babies for the first year. Yes, it's not uncommon; in fact, sharing a bed with your baby is not only common in many cultures but also has been practiced for millennia.

According to Dr. William Sears, the best way to foster positive sleep associations is to keep your baby right next to you in bed, preferably skin to skin when they're infants. Part of the philosophy behind co-sleeping is baby can feed on demand. You don't need to force baby to give up nighttime feedings or to sleep through the night.

This arrangement worked for me and my husband. We were all finally getting sleep. I set up a basket with a change pad, diapers, and wipes by my bed. Diaper changes happened right on the bed so I wouldn't even have to get up. Once my boys were six months old, it was easier to breastfeed at night. My baby would be curled up in my arm, and once he'd awaken, I'd slip up my top and offer my breast. It was effortless, and we'd both fall back asleep.

The thing is, you're so in tune with your baby that once you feel him rousing from sleep, you're also up. Although you're sleeping, you're aware of his presence. There was never a fear of rolling over him or falling off the bed either. Co-sleeping felt natural to me. Looking back now, it still was the best decision for our family. I treasure those extra cuddles during the night.

Research shows that babies who co-sleep may be at less risk for SIDS than babies who sleep alone.[61] If you choose to co-sleep, safety should be the top concern—and make sure your husband is on board! Read up on co-sleeping—including the pros and cons—and talk to your doctor before making this decision.

Co-sleeping is not for everyone, and there are some health concerns associated with co-sleeping.

Please note that the American Academy of Pediatrics recommends that "infants should sleep in the same bedroom as their parents—but on a separate surface, such as a crib or bassinet, and never on a couch, armchair, or soft surface—to decrease the risks of sleep-related deaths including sudden infant death syndrome or SIDS."[62]

AAP Recommendations on Creating a Safe Sleep Environment

- Place the baby on his or her back on a firm sleep surface such as a crib or bassinet with a tight-fitting sheet.
- Avoid use of soft bedding, including crib bumpers, blankets, pillows, and soft toys. The crib should be bare.
- Share a bedroom with parents, but not the same sleeping surface, preferably until the baby turns one but at least for the first six months. Room-sharing decreases the risk of SIDS by as much as 50 percent.
- Avoid baby's exposure to smoke, alcohol, and illicit drugs.[63]

While every baby and every parent is different, using good sleep practices and being patient—*super* patient—will help baby and mommy get the sleep they need. You won't be sleep deprived forever. You won't be stuck in the perpetual blur for all eternity! When you're in the thick of the newborn phase as a first-time mom, it's tough to see beyond the sleepless nights and barely-functioning days. But as time passes and baby grows, your sleep patterns will slowly return back to normal.

Sleep Deprived—For Years

This is a blog post I wrote when my second child was almost a year old and my firstborn was three years old. The title says it all.

Blog: Tired

January 18, 2008

I'm tired. Actually, I'm exhausted. The Underboss, my second child, is still waking up at night. Not just once or twice—I could handle that! I'm talking four, five, maybe six times a night. He is almost a year old.

I know I have to break his habit of night waking and nursing. I'm trying to wean him from breastfeeding and feel I'm making a bit of progress. But the problem is at night. Most of the time, the only way to get him back to sleep is to nurse him.

It's always felt very natural to nurse him to sleep. He's never taken to a bottle or pacifier, not even a stuffed animal. I tried teaching him how to suck his thumb like my first son, but he refused. When he was younger, he found comfort in snuggling up to a blanket, but now he only wants to snuggle up to my boobs.

I can't use the Ferber method—I can't do it! It's a personal choice. I'm an Attachment Parenting believer, because it's what feels natural to me, and I always like to go with my instinct.

I found Elizabeth Pantley's book The No-Cry Sleep Solution *very helpful, and I'm still trying the techniques on the Underboss. I used them on the Boss, and they did work. You have to be very persistent, and it takes several weeks to see results.*

I pick my battles with my boys, and sleep isn't really one of them. I don't have a problem helping my children fall asleep! I know some of you might be gasping in horror and pointing your finger with a "tisk tisk." I know some books and experts say you should let babies learn to fall asleep on their own. Yes, of course I'm doing the whole bedtime routine thing, but it's obviously not working. It did when my kids were infants . . . before they learned to manipulate!

What better place is there for a baby to fall asleep than in the arms of their Mommy or Daddy where it's warm and secure? When the Underboss wakes up during the night, I love taking him into bed with me, and I'll nurse him back to sleep most of the time. Once he dozes off, I'll wait about ten minutes until I know he's entered a good sleep phase and then sneak him back into his crib.

I have no problem with co-sleeping. I did it with the Boss, and for some reason it worked out well for a while, but with the Underboss, I find I can't sleep well at all. While you're thinking, Oh, you should get him to sleep in his OWN bed, I'm thinking, I should invest in a king-size bed.

There was a time when the Underboss would sleep six hours straight and I was able to get a nice deep sleep. But around six months, he started waking up every two hours again. Teething was at fault, but it became a habit.

The Boss would pop his thumb in his mouth to soothe himself, but he would still wake up at night. His sleep patterns really improved after he turned two and could sleep for nine hours. Does this mean I have to wait another year or so before I can get a full night's sleep? Arrrggh! In the meantime, I'll put the pot on, make another cup of coffee to keep me going, and dream of the day when my kids are teenagers and sleeping in until eleven o'clock in the morning!

But when that day comes, I know I'll think back and remember when my babies woke up at night and wanted me to hold them . . . I know I will miss those cuddly nights . . . so for now, I'm going to enjoy and cherish them while I can.

Chapter Thirteen

BABY'S MILESTONES

Developmental Milestones

The first year of a child's life is amazing to witness. From a helpless infant to an unstoppable toddler, in just twelve short months, your baby undergoes amazing changes and reaches many milestones. Babies grow at a remarkable pace, and every month brings astounding new developments.

It's normal for new parents to worry about baby's health and development, whether he is growing as he's supposed to and reaching those milestones on time. Don't worry if your child is the same age as another baby but hasn't reached the same milestones yet. Remember that babies develop at different rates, so if your baby has not reached one or more of these milestones, it does not mean that something is wrong. He or she will probably develop these skills within the next few months.

By around two months of age, your baby will smile in response to you! No, it's not gas this time—it's a real smile! The sound of your voice or the sight of your face is all it takes for your baby to start to smile. It's the most precious reward after the first few weeks of crying, feeding, and changing diapers.

By four months, that sweet little grin will turn into the cutest laughter. You'll have the best time making silly faces, tickling baby's feet, and playing peek-a-boo—anything to hear your baby's giggles and squeals. Just wait till baby discovers his hands and feet and those chubby little toes make their way into his mouth. Have the camera ready when this happens, which will likely be in the bathtub or during a diaper change. You'll love the way baby will suck on his toes!

By four to six months, some babies are capable of sleeping through the night (if you're lucky). Baby is also rolling over and spending time exploring on his tummy. Most babies can sit up with support by five or six months, either by resting on their hands in front of them or by leaning on pillows or furniture. When baby sits up for the very first time on his own, you're entering new baby cuteness territory! It's such a delight to see baby sitting up and reaching for and playing with new toys. It's a whole new perspective for him too, since he has spent so much time on his back or tummy.

Before baby begins crawling, you must childproof your home so that baby can explore and discover without the possibility of getting hurt. Make sure to install plug covers and baby gates as well as protect baby from sharp corners and breakable objects. You may consider hiring a professional baby-proofer to ensure your home is prepared for baby.

By nine months, most babies are crawling using both hands and feet. Along with crawling comes a newfound sense of independence for a baby. They are amazed by their own movement and proud of their accomplishments—especially if it's knocking down a block tower or throwing a spoon off their high chair over and over again!

Some babies never crawl but creep or move around on their bums instead! I remember feeling worried that my baby wasn't yet crawling. He would scoot around on his little bum and pull himself onto any piece of furniture he could find. Both of my boys liked to practice their quick movements, especially when I had my back turned for a split second. I would literally look away for a moment, look back, and find my baby had moved from sitting on the play mat to grabbing my feet. I'd look down, see his smiling face looking up at me, and know I was in serious trouble!

Before you know it, your baby will begin to make the link between sounds, gestures, and their meanings at the nine-month mark. Babies at this age can communicate by pointing, crawling, or gesturing toward desired objects. They can follow simple commands, like "give me the ball." They can also initiate and play gesture games, such as peek-a-boo and pat-a-cake. By this time too, they understand the meaning of "no." This is when the fun begins!

The best part of parenting this age is hearing baby say "Mama" or "Dada" for the very first time. Most babies are saying their first words by the time they turn one. Hearing those words will make your heart melt. You'll feel a sense of real accomplishment when you finally see your child communicate with you with words.

By twelve months, most babies begin to stand briefly without support, cruise while holding onto furniture, or even walk. You'll be amazed by how much your baby has grown and developed in just a short twelve months. This first year happens so quickly. Try to enjoy every age and stage. It won't be long before you finally get to see baby running!

Mom's Milestones

While baby is reaching important milestones, so are you! After six weeks, your uterus is back to normal and the swelling will have dissipated. Hopefully your body has recovered from childbirth, whether vaginal or C-section.

By two to three months, breastfeeding should be much easier. You'll have learned all the nursing positions and mastered holding your baby like a football too! Baby is latching on properly and sucking so effectively that you can finish a session within ten minutes on each side. You can handle a breast pump as efficiently as texting with one finger.

After the third month, baby's crying will have settled down, and you'll recognize what his cries mean and respond quickly. You're now a burping, feeding, diapering pro! You'll feel less sleep deprived as baby is sleeping better at night. At this point, you've also ditched the grandma panties and graduated back into that hot silky red number you normally save for date night.

By the fourth month, you'll have mastered getting yourself and baby ready for outings—packed and out the door within fifteen minutes! You'll hopefully have taken baby outside for stroller walks and found your favorite trail routes. Maybe you have joined a mom-and-baby salsa group and made new friends. Likely, you have even left baby for an hour or two with your hubby, mom, friend, or sitter to get to the gym!

By the fifth and sixth month, you're packing away your maternity jeans, as you now can fit back into your regular ones . . . or you may still opt for yoga pants! As you head to the grocery store, you might feel inclined to wear some makeup and let your hair down instead of sticking with your regular mom bun.

As soon as baby can sit up on his own, he can sit in the grocery cart! You will celebrate this milestone too because you will enjoy shopping much more now that baby will be a part of the fun. He will love looking at all of the colorful fruits and vegetables and cruising up and down the aisles. You will be discovering all the stores and shopping malls that have carts; IKEA, Home Depot, Target, and T. J. Maxx are all easy to navigate with baby in the cart seat. Who knew that would become so important!

At this point, you'll hopefully have had a date night with your partner or a mom's night out with your girlfriends. You'll also be a master juggler and multitasker; you can feed baby while talking on the phone and lifting weights to keep those triceps firm!

About midway through the first year, you will be feeling much more confident about yourself as a mother and your ability to care for baby and still feel quite human. It's truly amazing how much you've learned in the past six months!

Comparing Babies

Imagine a group of ten babies, all six months old. Some will be sitting steady, while others will be toppling over. One may be on her back, while another is almost ready to crawl.

If you have family or friends with babies, you'll be hearing a lot of comparing. It's inevitable; someone will at some point compare your baby to theirs or someone else's. Each baby is unique and develops at his own rate.

You may hear comments on how big or small your baby is or whether your baby has started sitting up or rolling over yet. No two babies are alike! As long as your baby is healthy and thriving, you can rest assured that they'll grow up just fine.

Babies vary widely when it comes to hitting the big milestones like sitting up, crawling, and walking. As parents, we're encouraged to watch for any development delays and to talk to the doctor about our concerns. While baby development charts are helpful, some parents seem to focus on and worry too much about specific dates. While some babies may reach certain milestones on the earlier side, others will be closer to the later range.

"Oh, my baby is already sitting up at three months!"

Comparing a child's development with other children is natural. It's when parents become competitive that it becomes troublesome. Competitive parents see early development as a sign of intelligence, good parenting, and superstardom. Just because their baby is rolling over front to back to front at four months doesn't mean he's going to be a famous gymnast. Each baby has his own developmental pace; reaching milestones on the early side or "ahead of schedule" doesn't indicate top IQ scores and the gifted program at school down the road.

You must know at least one perfectionist parent who brags incessantly about her baby who reached every milestone early. Oh yes, that baby is going to be a genius because he said more than five words by the age of eleven months and was already running before the age of one. There was one mom in particular who I felt tried to one-up me any chance she could get. If I mentioned how excited I was that my son rolled over finally, she would gloat that her baby did that a month ago. She did the exact same thing when I announced how exciting it was to see the Boss sitting up and playing with his toys for the first time. She scoffed and included the fact that her son did the same thing when he was only five months old.

Once you've completed rolling your eyes and vowing never to arrange a playdate with that mom, try not to focus too much on those development milestones, and remember that all babies develop at their own pace.

"I have such a good baby!"

Because baby eats well, sleeps well, and rarely cries, often parents will describe their baby as being an "easy" or "good" baby. So if your baby doesn't fit the description of a "good" baby, does that make him or her bad? Of course not! There are babies who can be described as "fussy" or "high needs," which means that they may be more challenging to parent.

My first baby would feed constantly and never nap. He also cried for three hours a day for the first three months. He wasn't the greatest sleeper; he slept near me, or with me, waking often. When I'd hear other moms say that their two-month-old was sleeping six hours straight a night, I was baffled. Some babies sleep like a dream, while others fight bedtime with every ounce of strength in their tiny bodies. *Is my baby the only one who cries a lot and doesn't sleep?* I thought I was the only one who had these challenges as a new mom. But then when I started talking to other moms, I soon realized that most were just as frustrated as I was.

Each one of us had our own set of challenges; while my baby wasn't the best napper, he loved trying different solid foods. While a friend's baby slept through the night, she was a nightmare during car rides. Do your best to let comparisons fly and just love on your baby.

Comparing Moms

Not only will moms compare their babies, they will compare themselves too. When you become a mother, you don't become a mother of all; you become the mother of your own children. No one can parent your child the way you can, and no mother can do a better job raising your kids than you.

Babies don't come with instructions—I wish they did! Moms (and dads) have to make decisions about their children every day, and often they question those decisions, wondering whether they made the best choices.

The stress associated with this huge responsibility can be overwhelming at times! The result is that moms feel they have to justify their parenting choices to anyone who questions them.

When a mom convinces herself that her way is the right or best way, she can then enter competitive territory where she may judge others for their parenting style and their lifestyle choices. Even if you're not judging another mom in a negative manner, you still may find yourself comparing.

This happens when we squeeze ourselves into a type of mom category . . . stay-at-home mom, working mom, breastfeeding mom, to name a few. It's human nature to want to fit in somewhere, whether it's the mainstream norm or another particular group. When views and choices don't fit that norm, some women are left feeling discouraged and subpar.

How can I measure up to what other moms are doing?

Wow, that mom is grocery shopping with her baby in high heels! How does she have time to do her nails and makeup?!

You may be scratching your head wondering how *that mom* managed to lose all of her baby weight in a month while you're still struggling seven months later. You may see a mom who seems to be super organized and looks put together; you may then feel worse about yourself because your hair is in a mom bun, you have no makeup on, and you're still wearing your maternity jeans.

Even online, when you scroll through Facebook or Instagram, you might see other moms who seem to have it all together. Most of the time, social media shows just a snapshot (which is likely staged) of their life. Every day, we see images and read stories that leave us feeling as if every parent is doing it better than we are.

If social media is making you feel less confident, stop scrolling. You need to ignore how other moms are doing it and focus on what works for you. Those picture-perfect moments are not reality; they are just an image of a single moment. If you can remember that behind every seemingly ideal photo is a mom who feels just like you do, you'll be much better off.

When looking at other moms, it's important to keep things in perspective and be inspired by differences. Instead of beating yourself up, focus on your strengths and be grateful for what you have and can do!

We all have moments of low self-esteem or insecurity—it's completely normal! But we can change that inner dialogue to tell ourselves that we ARE good enough. Be secure in your own decisions. When we feel good about our own decisions, we feel less of a need to justify our actions. Give yourself a pep talk, just as you would to a friend. Remind yourself that you've got this!

Growth Spurts

I thought I had this parenting gig down pat. Then my baby went through a growth spurt.

Once you feel like you're into a groove: "I've got this motherhood thing—oh yeah!" and you have a new sense of confidence and surge of self-esteem about your mothering, BOOM. A shift happens. Suddenly your baby wants your boob or the bottle nonstop. "Didn't I just feed you?"

Oh yes, the growth spurts. Babies go through quite a few of them in the first year: at around ten days, three weeks, six weeks, three months, and six months. I don't even mean growth as in weight gain, while of course it's amazing to see the poundage pack on and those folding rolls develop on their legs! Baby is suddenly getting longer—growing right out of that favorite sleeper. Believe me; you will notice!

Dr. Martha and William Sears of *The Breastfeeding Book* say to think of these as "frequency days" when babies want and need to nurse all the time because they are growing very quickly. You'll be "marathon nursing" for a day or two until your body produces more milk, and then baby will need to feed less often.[64] Baby is demanding more milk, and your body is working hard to supply it! That's when you start to feel like you should throw a cowbell around your neck and call yourself Bertha the Moo Moo.

Babies' brains are growing, too, and they're learning about the world around them as they reach all those physical milestones like rolling over, sitting up, and crawling. According to *What to Expect the First Year*, babies who are sleeping through the night can have setbacks; for example, if they are cutting a tooth, going through a change of routine, or even celebrating a milestone like rolling over or standing up, they may wake up more in the night.[65]

Teething was a major cause of utter disruption and frustration when my boys were about five and six months old. It doesn't take much to turn a baby's routine on its head. A cold or an ear infection can wreak havoc on sleeping patterns too. Also, a change in routine—for example, traveling or mom returning to work—can temporarily interfere with established sleep patterns.

What can you do to get through these trying times? Camp out on the couch with the remote control or Netflix, some herbal tea, and a stash of chips and chocolate because you'll be tied down for a while. Comfort your distressed babe through these disruptions in her schedule.

Don't worry; you'll be back into your groove again soon. Be comforted by the fact that this is a phase. It won't last forever. My mantra for a long time was *This too shall pass*. Tattoo it on your wrist or, if you are the crafty type, embroider it on your pillow.

Mom Challenges Are Real

As you watch your baby reach these remarkable milestones, there will be days when you're so exhausted and frustrated. Like when the baby has been screaming for over an hour and nothing seems to settle him down, you may find yourself daydreaming about being back at work or, even better, hopping on a plane for the Caribbean sands and surf.

While you realize you're lucky to be home with the baby, you can't feel grateful every moment. Not everything you do with baby is going to feel #blessed. When you stub your toe on the way to pick up a hungry baby in the middle of the night, you're not going to be thinking, *Oh, motherhood is so great.* You won't be praising the joys of motherhood when you're cleaning up baby's third diaper explosion. There are going to be crappy moments along with the sweet, memorable ones—and that's perfectly okay.

Some days you'll look around and, though you smile at your beaming baby who is beginning to coo, your eyes will catch the pile of dishes in the kitchen sink. You didn't expect to be constantly washing, cleaning, changing diapers, and feeding 24/7.

I don't think we fully understand all the work that goes into being a parent until we actually become one. There is no practice for motherhood, no dress rehearsal. You just go through it, one step at a time, and learn as you go along. If you come to accept that you will make mistakes along the way and do the best that you can, you will do just fine.

There are some remarkable, amazing moments that first year of baby's life; others you would not mind forgetting. But through it all, there is nothing else you would rather do than be a mother to your baby. The moment you look into baby's eyes, your heart melts and all the challenges don't mean a thing! Watching this little human being grow, smile, giggle, and reach out for you makes everything worthwhile.

Chapter Fourteen

BABY WILL ALWAYS BE HUNGRY AND CLINGY

"I'm hungry!"

For the first few months, feeding baby is a breeze. Breast milk is the number one option for nutrition and convenience. Baby's hungry? Sure, I'll just pop out my breast and she can chow down! For women who don't or can't breastfeed, formula is convenient and anyone can feed baby. Grandma would be thrilled to take over so Mama can take a hot shower.

There's nothing cuter than a newborn that is rooting for Mama's nipple. What a cute yet cruel little joke to tease baby—you must try it at least once—but not for long; otherwise she will snap her mouth at your sore nipples like a crocodile chomping on a fish.

Once baby reaches the milestone of beginning to eat solid foods, it's a whole new world of flavor and taste. This is when you can also be a big meanie and look forward to offering citrus fruits like lemons—make sure to have your finger on the record button for that event!

If your baby spits out what you offer her, there may be a reason. I can't get angry at baby for spitting out the mashed green beans with absolutely no salt or seasoning—can you blame the child? How would you like it if you were served bland and boring chicken puree with peas?!

Cereals, vegetables, fruits . . . babies will explore food and drool, spit, and make a mess while they experiment with their palates. It's another milestone that you will get a kick out of watching. Keep a food journal so you can document whether baby loved it or hated the new food and if she suffered any negative reaction. Give the new food a few days before determining whether the food isn't causing any gas, bloating, and/or changes in bowel movements.

If you notice any signs of allergy, record this too and don't offer that food again until you get the okay from your doctor. Sometimes doctors will recommend waiting up to a year before trying that food again. Other times you will be advised to stay away from that food for life.

When Is Baby Ready to Start Solids?

Human milk or commercial formula alone will meet the nutritional needs of infants up to age six months. After that, solid foods are needed to augment energy sources and provide adequate vitamins and iron. The American Academy of Pediatrics (AAP) recommends starting solids no earlier than age four months.

Feeding solids before age four months may result in aspiration and is associated with a slightly increased risk of developing obesity, type 1 diabetes, and celiac disease. Waiting until significantly later than age six months can result in inadequate energy intake, leading to slow growth, disinterest in solid foods, delayed oropharyngeal motor development, and iron deficiency. Be aware of your baby's cues. If there is any doubt, consult your doctor.

Begin introducing solids when your baby is developmentally ready—for example, when he has good head and neck control and when he's able to sit with support. When baby is ready, he will no longer be pushing out material placed between his lips. He'll also communicate interest in food by leaning forward and opening his mouth. Often baby will start eyeing the food on Mom's and Dad's plates. This is a cue that he is curious and may be ready for solids.

Every baby is different, and the amount that your baby eats can change from day to day. Your baby may also eat more or less than other babies. Your baby will let you know when he is full. It may take many attempts for your baby to accept a new food. This is common! If your baby doesn't like the new food, you can try offering the food again in a few days.

According to the American Academy of Pediatrics, single-grain cereals are usually introduced to baby first. If you do start with cereal, make sure it's made for babies and is iron fortified. But you can offer vegetables or meat first if you wish. Many pediatricians will recommend starting vegetables before fruits since babies are born with a preference for sweets. Breastfeeding babies may benefit from starting with meats, which contain more easily absorbed sources of iron and zinc that are needed by four to six months of age.

Here are some tips to consider:

- Start by offering food two to three times a day and work toward three to five times a day. Consider two to three meals and one to two snacks each day based on their appetite. Your baby will decide how much she wants to eat.
- Start with a small amount, such as one teaspoon. If your baby shows you that she wants more food, give her more.

- Start with soft foods that have been pureed, mashed, minced, or ground, and as baby gets older, introduce lumpier foods and finger foods.
- It's super easy to prepare your own baby food; just cook fruits and vegetables until soft and then use a blender or food processor to puree, chop, and blend. You can just mash softer foods with the back of a fork. Don't use salt or seasonings.
- Be sure to refrigerate any leftover food and use within one to two days.
- Do not give your baby any food that can be a choking hazard, including hot dogs, nuts and seeds, large chunks of meat or cheese, whole grapes or large fruit chunks, raw vegetables, or candy.
- Introduce new foods one at a time and wait two to three days before offering another new food. It helps to keep a food journal of what your baby is sampling, whether she likes it or not, and if she has any reactions.

First Foods

At six to eight months, you can offer iron-rich foods such as:
- Well-cooked pureed, mashed, finely minced, or shredded meat, poultry, or fish, including beef, pork, chicken, turkey, cod, and halibut
- Well-cooked mashed eggs, tofu, lentils, or beans
- Iron-fortified infant cereals such as oatmeal, barley, or rice mixed with breast milk or infant formula
- Well-cooked mashed sweet potato and squash
- Soft-cooked pieces of broccoli and carrots
- Well-cooked mashed mango, pears, peaches, and banana
- Plain cottage cheese and yogurt

Continue to offer breast milk. Baby will be ready for finger foods when she can pick up objects with her thumb and forefinger, can transfer items from one hand to another, and can move her jaw in a chewing motion. This usually occurs around eight to ten months.

At eight to ten months, you can also offer:

- O-shaped cereal
- Small well-cooked pieces of vegetables and fruit
- Well-cooked pasta like rotini or penne
- Small pieces of scrambled eggs, meat, or fish
- Small pieces of toast or bagel
- Teething crackers
- Grated cheddar, mozzarella, and swiss cheese

You can also introduce baby to sips of water in an open cup, but do not let your baby fill up on water.

By ten to twelve months, baby will have more teeth and can eat more foods! You will now be able to ditch the blender and allow baby's food to have more texture. Offer soft or cooked fruit cut into cubes or strips and bite-size, soft-cooked vegetables as well as small pieces of meat, poultry, boneless fish, and well-cooked beans. Chop all foods into soft, bite-size pieces one-half inch or smaller.

Sample Meals for a 10- to 12-Month-Old

Breakfast	• Iron-fortified infant cereal or chopped egg • Mashed banana or shredded apple
Snack	• Whole grain crackers with shredded cheddar

Lunch	• Minced chicken breast or mashed chickpeas with mashed sweet potato • Yogurt and chopped kiwi
Snack	• Mashed pear or chopped soft cantaloupe
Dinner	• Ground beef, fish, or lentils with brown rice, mashed and cooked broccoli • Unsweetened applesauce

Picky Eater

My firstborn would devour any vegetable puree I whipped up. Well, mostly any. You see, even babies have a preference for certain flavors and foods. Mashed bananas and cooked apples: delicious! Carrots and peas were gone within seconds. Fillet of fish gobbled up while my husband and I looked on in pure shock. But green beans? Blech! Chicken? No way!

Your baby will let you know if she doesn't like a certain food. She may push away the spoon or turn her head away. She may clamp her mouth tightly shut as you try to feed her. If the Boss didn't like a new food, he would just spit it out, cringing and shivering as if he had just sucked on a lemon.

Here are some tips for the picky eater:

- Keep offering your baby healthy and wholesome foods. Don't force it, though; if baby is growing and healthy, don't worry. Baby will let you know when they've finished eating.
- Try introducing one new flavor a week. Offering variety prepares her for a balanced diet down the road.
- Try combining a food baby loves with a food they usually refuse. It's a good trick! Then gradually increase the flavor of the food they first disliked.

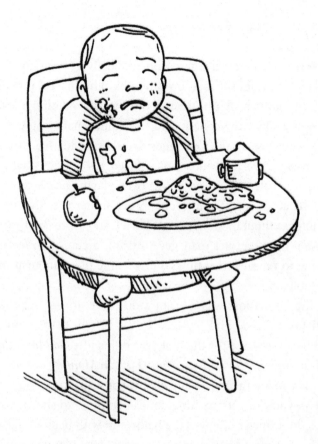

- Why not spice things up? Add some seasoning such as cinnamon or garlic to give a little kick to their meals. But don't reach for added sugar, salt, or flavors with preservatives.
- Let baby touch the food! There are few creatures more hands on than a baby. Let him touch and swish those pureed pears. Baby may want to fully experience his food before he puts it in his mouth.
- Start eating alongside baby. Once baby begins solids, you can start having family meals together.

"I'm clingy!"

After surviving a challenging labor and delivery with my firstborn, and then colic for the first three months of his life, I was ready for a normal routine. After he turned four months old, things started to get easier. Once the colic subsided, I could finally enjoy him. The Boss would be awake for longer stretches, didn't have to be held and rocked every minute, and enjoyed his bouncy chair, swing, and baby mat. He enjoyed rolling over, playing on his tummy, and looking at his toys. I could actually get dinner prepared in twenty minutes without interruption. What a feat! Before this time, it was a *really good* day if I managed to drink a cup of coffee without having to reheat it two times and get an edible, unburnt meal on the table.

The Underboss was a bit of a different story . . . he was ON TOP OF ME ALL THE TIME. He wanted to be held, sit on my lap, and be all over me for the first year of his life. *God bless that cute little pumpkin, I love him to death, but can Mommy just pee alone?!* When you are raising a clingy baby, you tend to get very creative just so you can get anything done. You learn to shower with the glass door open and go to the bathroom with baby in his bouncy chair . . . you share moments you really never planned on sharing.

Blog: Apron Strings

June 2, 2008

One of the roughest weeks I had as a mom was when I got hit with another bout of mastitis. This time was the last straw. It was time to wean the Underboss. Unfortunately, this was a lot harder than I thought!

Rather than enjoying his new taste for a variety of foods, it seemed he wanted more and more milk. I'm sure it was more of the sucking that he wanted (he never took to a soother), but it was becoming ridiculous. The only way he would fall back asleep at night was to suckle at my breast. Although I still enjoyed breastfeeding, it was becoming clearer that it would be difficult to get him off my milk machines. To top it off, both boys caught a nasty virus, which gave them a fever, and since germs naturally gravitate toward me, I caught that too.

Amazing how the whole house can fall apart when Mommy is

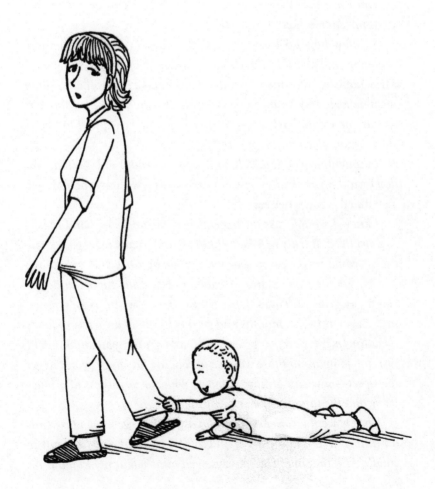

sick. The kids are confused because they see you lying on the couch rather than multitasking like a madwoman. Hubby doesn't know where to find the sugar. Did you move the peanut butter and look behind it? *This is the time when you really want your own mom to come over and make you a big pot of chicken soup.*

I had enough! I didn't want to wean, but it was time. The antibiotics I was used to taking for previous bouts were not strong enough this time and my doctor was unavailable, so I had to visit a walk-in clinic—I just love having my boobs poked and examined!

Did I mention that once the antibiotics finished, the wonderful yeast infection kicked in? Lovely!

So now, how do I gently break the news to the boob guzzler? "No more milk," I told the Underboss matter-of-factly. "All gone." Miraculously, he seemed to understand it. Like it was the headline news delivered by Walter Cronkite! No questions asked. I thought for sure he would have a meltdown every time he wanted to feed. I should have given him more credit.

I thought he would take it badly, but instead, I did. "What, you don't want my milk anymore?" What's wrong with my milk, dude? You like the cow's better?

I knew I would miss the dependence, the amazing bond that is so short lived. It truly is! Waahhhhh! I wasn't ready to let go. I knew that I would miss that special mommy-baby time. But you know, when your little one starts to playfully bite your nipple and give you a coy grin while he's doing it, it's time to wean. If he's eating up a storm at twelve months and getting his fill of a variety of foods including meat, dairy, veggies, fruits, and grains, your milk might just not compare to those wonderful cooking flavors! Try not to get too upset—how can a mom compete with the sweetness of a blueberry and the tartness of a crunchy apple? Sigh.

To replace the closeness from breastfeeding, we have more cuddle time. I need it and crave it and so does he—but now he wants to cuddle ALL the time! He's always been attached at my hip, but it's *become more extreme lately.*

My back is killing me, not from lifting weights to tone up my flabby arms . . . it's because I'm holding the Underboss all day long. No joke; most of the day I spend holding him in my arms. Over twenty-five pounds, clinging to me from morning until night. Some nights I'll have to bring him into my bed, and he will climb on top of me and fall back asleep. It's the cutest thing; in his tiny voice, he'll say "Hug," clutch onto me, and give me the biggest bear hug ever.

Now that the milk machines have retired, he has found another way to keep me by his side. And if I sway, even for a few minutes, he will freak.

If I just go to the front door to grab the newspaper, the Underboss comes running, crying "Mummyyyyy!!" A trip to the washroom can send him into panic mode, like I've left to never come back. Exits have to be really quick—no pausing for long goodbyes; a quick kiss and I'm out the door. He'll fuss and whine for a few minutes, but then he'll get distracted and be okay. But he will go back and forth to the front door, look out the window, and call for me, waiting for me to come home.

Don't get me wrong; I love that he wants me all the time. It's the best feeling in the world to see that little face beaming at me, running to me the moment I open the door. But this separation anxiety has lasted longer than I expected.

I'm sad that we no longer have the breastfeeding bond anymore . . . it's just another apron string that has been cut loose on my baby's way to independence. And although there are moments when I get frustrated by his clinginess, I know that one day in the near future, he'll be off and running and won't want to hold his Mommy every second. So, for the time being, I will try and cherish this time, because it'll be gone before I know it.

While baby will be always hungry and clingy, those first few months are the ones to cherish as much as possible because they do fly right by. It still amazes me to think about the milestones they reach in the early years. From a helpless infant to an energetic toddler, these are the times that we must hold near and dear. There is that truth that slams you right in the face: my baby will never be a baby again.

Chapter Fifteen

YOUR RELATIONSHIP WITH YOUR PARTNER WILL CHANGE

I f someone tells you that their relationship after baby didn't change, they're not being honest with you. For many couples, the relationship undergoes many changes when transitioning from a couple to a brand-new family. Baby makes three!

The first year of becoming parents is like a big test to see if your marriage can survive. If you make it through the first year as a couple, you can make it through anything! Think of this time as a challenge to be conquered, and realize that your marriage can emerge even stronger.

Before baby arrives, couples spend time getting the nursery ready, going to ultrasound appointments, and getting excited about baby's arrival. But couples don't typically talk about how things will change once the baby comes . . . usually because they don't quite realize how much will change. Once the baby arrives, much of the attention you were giving to each other is now focused on your baby. Your whole life revolves around this little person who needs your attention around the clock. This can leave one or both of you feeling lonely and neglected.

It's tough to give each other 100 percent of your attention when baby has so many needs. You don't have the time or energy you used to have—and some couples find that challenging. It's common for new parents to feel a distance between them.

If either of you are feeling exhausted, overlooked, or left out, it doesn't mean that your relationship is a failure—it simply means you just had a baby! It's going to take some time to find your new groove and think: *Okay; I've got this.* Once you get a handle on being new parents, the reconnection of your marriage will follow.

How You Might Be Feeling

If your partner goes back to work full time and you're home alone with the baby, you may begin to feel overwhelmed with different thoughts and emotions. Of course, you wouldn't trade this for the world. But your life has changed so much while his seems quite the same. He still gets to get up in the morning, get dressed, and go to work, where he'll interact and socialize with other adults. Meanwhile, you'll feel like you've been changing diapers, looking at the four walls of your house, and talking in a baby voice all day long!

From five o'clock to seven o'clock in the evening, or what we all call the witching hour, baby is fussy, cranky, and overtired, and you're starving, trying to put some food on the table. Dad gets home from work after a stressful day only to hear baby wailing and see an upside-down kitchen. Mom is ready to pass baby over to Dad, who just returned from a stressful day and wants a few minutes to himself. Mom is ready to scream. Dad is fit to be tied. When do parents get a break?

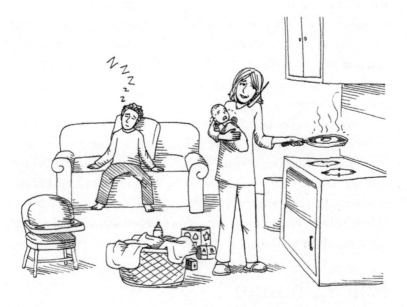

I remember feeling resentful that I was the one who had to endure hours of labor and a difficult childbirth. I was the one whose body underwent wacky yet miraculous changes and would have to deal with losing all that baby weight. I was the one who had to master breastfeeding and endure cracked and bleeding nipples. I resented that he could eat whatever he wanted but I had to watch what I ate because the foods I ingested might make baby gassy. He could take a long, hot shower, but I had to hurry to finish before baby awoke. Why did I have to sacrifice my body and my routine while my husband's stayed much the same?

It's very easy to feel a sense of loss of identity once the baby arrives. Everything is all about the baby! You won't have the time together that you used to have. Your weeknights will be more hectic than before kids, so it will take some adjusting, careful planning, and perhaps outside help (Babysitters!) to get into a routine.

You will come to realize that as parents, you each have different roles in the family unit. Talk with your partner; don't let tradition or media decide what will work best in your home. Be honest and open with yourself and each other. Discuss what works for each of you and your lifestyles, and make a plan together. Remember that your plan and roles may change over time, so flexibility and understanding are key.

Once you have settled into a bit of a schedule and you have a better handle on taking care of baby, you will have more time to focus on the two of you. You'll have to make time, and although it may seem like a huge effort sometimes, it's important for a healthy relationship. Your marriage is going to take a little bit of work to keep it healthy, functioning, and—don't forget—fun. It's time to set those wheels in motion.

Roles Change

Before your first child, you likely had a system in the house, a schedule and lists of tasks that each partner would be responsible for. All that is thrown out the window once baby arrives. You and your partner will need to work together to make a new system that works for your new family.

Good communication is really the key to creating good cooperation and a great family. Have a weekly meeting to sync your calendars. This helps avoid miscommunication and the resulting arguments, about, for example, who needs to work late—and who needs to be home with the baby. It may be worth dividing up who does what for the baby and the household. You may even need to break it down from paying bills and cooking dinner to getting up with the baby at three o'clock in the morning—write down who is going to be responsible for each task. But remember: life happens. Be flexible.

If you choose to be a stay-at-home mom, those roles and responsibilities may change even more.

"Well, since you're home, you have time to cook and clean." This is a huge misconception and one that needs to be remedied immediately. A mother's role is to take care of her baby and herself first and foremost. Then come the other household tasks—if there is sufficient time left. Some days you will have time to take care of those tasks, while other days you will have to let the laundry wait and order takeout. This is not a parenting fail—it is natural life, especially when baby is sick, teething, or fussy.

I often hear other women complain, "But why do I have to ask? He should just know!" While you may expect your spouse to instinctively be aware of what needs to be done with the baby or around the house, he may not. You may have to ask him nicely and delegate tasks. Communicate. Understand that he is not intentionally trying to piss you off. He may not discern your emotions—although abundantly clear to you—unless you simply tell him how you're feeling. *Even* then, he may not understand what he should be doing—be very clear in communicating what you need from him.

You may not feel you should have to give him precise instructions, but it may be just what he requires to help you. Likely he will greatly appreciate it. While you think he *should* know what you're thinking and feeling, he is most likely not a mind reader. So you may need to guide him.

Don't say "You're not helping enough around the house." Instead, say "It would really help me if you would take out the garbage every night before bed and empty the dishwasher." Or "It would really help me if you can clean up the kitchen after dinner and run the baby a bath. I could really use a half hour to myself to unwind because I'll likely be up a few times tonight to feed the baby. Thanks, honey."

Asking nicely and giving exact details on how you're feeling rather than blurting out your frustrations will benefit you both. While you may expect a big sigh from him, you'll be amazed when he replies "Okay." You'll wonder why you didn't speak to him like this a long time ago! *If it's that easy to get him to help me out, then I'll be sure to coat everything with sugar and extra sprinkles every time!*

As you go through the first weeks and months, use the weekly meeting to help communicate needs and make a plan. Be open to your partner's ideas and solutions. Guys love to solve a problem when they know there is one! Understand that there will be a lot of fine-tuning as you go along in this parenting adventure.

Taking Care of the Baby

Like new moms, new dads also need encouragement, reassurance, support, and to vent their worries and thoughts. Have open communication, and remember to support each other. Allow dad to help with the baby, and be patient with him. I remember how nervous my husband was the first time he changed baby's diaper—he nearly passed out from the color of baby's poop! Once we finished sharing a good laugh, the anxiety came back. He was anxious that he would hurt the baby or be too rough with him as he delicately pulled baby's little arms through the sleeper and snapped the buttons over baby's diaper. But after a few weeks with sufficient practice, he became super comfortable. Also, hubby enjoyed burping duty; the first time I showed him the technique where baby sits outward on your lap leaning slightly forward, with your hand supporting baby's jaw, he was scared to try it! But then when he burped baby over his shoulder and dribbled spit-up down his back, he was happy to try it again!

Some men are more in tune with their partners and take on the role of fatherhood naturally. But remember that the whole "natural mother" thing doesn't always happen to women either—keep in mind that we all have our struggles and preconceived notions—and then real life happens. There are some men who are more instinctually parental, while others seem to struggle with father-hood. Rather than becoming frustrated and angry at your partner, it's helpful to know that this new role will take some practice and plenty of support from you!

Give your spouse a chance to practice swaddling or bathing the baby and *take a step back*. It's the Mama Bear in us that pushes us to step in when, really, we should be supportive and allow him to do things himself. I learned to let go of the reins so he could take charge, which was best for both of us—and baby too. I promise baby will survive and love her papa all the more.

Night Shift

Dads can help with feeding baby during the night, giving baby and Daddy precious alone time. If mom is nursing, he can still help; while he can't breastfeed, he can help you get comfortable while you nurse. You can pump your milk and Dad can feed the baby while you sleep. He may not have the instincts to wake up as easily when the baby cries in the middle of the night, but he can sleep closest to the bassinet so he can wake up and help out with the late-night feedings. If baby is formula-fed, you can alternate feeding times so that you're both getting sleep.

Come to a compromise that will benefit the both of you, and keep in mind that if he's at the office, it will be harder for him to sneak an afternoon nap than it may be for you. The work my hus-band does can be dangerous, so it's important for him to be extra alert during the day. Concerned about him having a good night's sleep and his safety, I wouldn't allow him to wake to help during the night. As with any parenting choice, keep an open mind and decide what works best for your family!

Diaper Duty

Your partner can also change baby's diaper during the night or anytime to give Mama a break. He may have two left hands and fumble when changing baby, but give him time to get comfortable with the baby—he'll be a pro sooner than you think.

Cuddle and Soothe

Dad can rock baby, walk her around, and soothe her when she's crying. Baby can also learn that Mommy isn't the only one who can make her feel better. There are plenty of babies out there who love to nuzzle into Dad's arms and hear his deep voice. I noticed a huge shift in the baby-daddy relationship during the second half of baby's first year; while I dominated the newborn phase when it came to cuddle time, Dad reigned supreme in the second half.

Sing Songs

Okay, maybe your spouse doesn't have a great voice, but baby won't care! Whether he sings a lullaby or rocks out to Foo Fighters, Dad can provide hours of silly entertainment.

Take Baby for a Walk

Nice day outside? Let Daddy take baby for a walk and enjoy some fresh air. He can push baby in a stroller or keep her close in a sling or carrier while Mom has a moment to herself. Ahhh.

Playtime

Set aside time every day for playtime—after dinner or before bedtime begins. Baby will begin to look forward to the routine! Dad can make silly faces, play gentle bouncy games, cuddle, and tickle and even play peek-a-boo when baby is older.

Bedtime Routine

Daddy can be a part of the bedtime routine by helping with bath time or reading a book. Dad can also give baby massages. This may prepare him to give Mom one too—oh, the benefits!

Building Your Relationship Must Be a Priority

After going through the difficult sleep-deprivation phase and getting into the groove of being a mom while watching your partner gain some awesome dad skills, the feeling of empowerment takes over. *Wow, I've embraced my powerful abilities as a woman—after all, I can give birth and breastfeed like a pro!* That is truly remarkable. Your partner will have ninja diaper-changing skills and be able to burp baby on command. He knows just the right bouncy rhythm baby likes to soothe his cries. He's come to realize that there will be days when you just want to spend some time alone while he cares for baby. You may even decide to buy matching Awesome Mom/Dad t-shirts—high fives all around!

Now that you've moved into your new roles in your family unit, it's time to shift your focus back toward each other. A little bit of effort can go a long way.

Thank Each Other

Giving thanks is the simplest and most appreciated thing you can do to your partner. Your spouse leaves your bundle of joy each day to go to work—thank him. If Hubby is on night duty to feed baby—thank him. For dads, if Mom is breastfeeding exclusively—thank her for that. Remind each other that you matter and that you are loved for who you are, not just what you do.

Make Time for Each Other

Even though you may not have the energy after a long day to talk, or one of you falls asleep before the other, schedule in some time for the two of you to connect. It could be as simple as a few cuddles on the sofa or sitting down together for dinner.

Plan a date night—this could mean going out literally or simply carving out some time after baby is down for the night (at least for now). Even watching a funny movie together and having some laughs can be all it takes to rekindle the romance. The key is to *plan*—remember those weekly meetings? They aren't just to assign jobs. You can plan a romantic couple's night together, which sends a message that your marriage is important too (see more on date nights later in this chapter).

What Sex Life?

> *New dads need to understand that when ten o'clock rolls around, exhausted mom would prefer to be sleeping—they shouldn't expect a black lace lingerie and red patent-leather heels in the bedroom.*

It's no secret that the birth of a child can be a challenge for many couples as they undergo a transition from a couple to a family. One common finding in studies of parental relationships is that parents report a decrease in satisfaction in their marital relationship right after baby is born, as well as a year or even several years after baby. After having a baby, marital quality decreases precipitously in 40 to 67 percent of married couples beginning within the first year of the baby's life.[66] There are many factors that play a role, including gender roles, parental expectations, division of the workload, financial stress, and even the strength of the relationship before baby.

The transition affects couples in positive and negative ways. "On the positive side, parents often experience a sense of gratification and joy over having a new baby. On the negative side, they may also experience exhaustion, lack of time for themselves, and more disagreement over issues pertaining to care of the baby and the division of family labor. These strains and difficulties may affect the quality of their relationship as a couple adversely."[67]

Many couples just don't talk about it! They ease into their new roles—she as new mother, he as new father—and lose the wife-husband relationship as they become parents to their offspring. At some point, however, you will need to focus on your relationship again.

Keep in mind that having a child doesn't necessarily mean a couple is more likely to split; in one study, the divorce rate was 50 percent for couples who remained childless compared to a divorce rate of 25 percent for couples who became parents.[68] Regardless of whether research suggests having a baby decreases marital satisfaction, strengthening the marriage is something couples need to focus on post-baby, whether on their own, through professional programs, or therapy.

Ease Back into Sex

Your boobs are leaking, you're carrying extra weight everywhere, and you now have a lovely pooch and stretch marks. Not feeling so desirable, and after only a few hours of sleep, changing diapers, and getting spit up on, the last thing you feel like doing is pleasing your husband. You are thinking, *When do I get a break?!?* Your husband is throwing you a sultry look, while you have dark circles under your eyes, your hair is half up, and you're ready to WRING HIS NECK! You are so not in the mood.

After our firstborn came into our lives, the six weeks postpartum felt much longer. I had badly torn and was still sore after the six-week mark. There was no way he was going anywhere near me. I was scared to have sex again, to be honest—I was afraid it would be painful. Let's just say it didn't feel quite right down there for some time. If you have continuing pain, talk to your doctor. Your relationship is worth it!

I didn't feel desirable either—my body was much *softer* than it had ever been. I was still wearing maternity jeans past the three-month postpartum mark. I was lucky if I had taken a shower in the last twenty-four hours. I was pretty much living in sweatpants and spit-up-stained shirts. I definitely didn't feel sexy—go figure.

Once the chaos of the newborn phase has passed, the colic has subsided, the baby is sleeping more than three hours at a time, and you're *almost* feeling human again, you'll want to have some intimacy with your spouse—right? For some women, sex is that last thing on your mind. It's true that you're getting a ton of cuddles with your baby and enjoying that physical closeness. But at some point, you'll want to save some snuggles for Hubby.

Dads who are working full time aren't able to enjoy that physical contact as much as moms do. Many hubbies feel a lack of love and intimacy. They feel left out because all of Mom's attention is showered on the baby. And they still want to have sex with you. You may not be interested in making him feel loved, because you're so darn tired all the time. You care, but you are drained or maybe even touched out and need space. The day-to-day grind can get in the way of any romance, so you'll have to make the effort now more than ever before.

Common Excuses for Not Being in the Mood

- I'm tired.
- I don't want any more skin-to-skin contact.
- I'm mad at him.
- I have a million things to do.
- The baby is going to wake any second.
- Not in front of the baby!

How to Combat These Reasons and Get into the Mood

- Try to take an afternoon nap so you have a little more energy in the evening.
- Get baby to bed before eight o'clock (this may take months).
- Start slow—maybe you don't go *all the way* your first time after giving birth (it's okay).
- Have a sense of humor—the baby may wake. Laugh it off and try again later.
- If you are mad at hubby, kiss and make up and . . . you know . . .

- You may be very wound up; take some deep breaths, ask for a nice massage, and see where that goes.
- What put you in the mood before baby? Try nice music, a bubble bath . . .
- Send each other sexy text messages during the day to increase the excitement.
- Who said sex happens only at night? Try morning or afternoon during baby's nap.
- Realize that sex is important too—put it on the to-do list.

Spouses are more likely to get lucky if they help with baby care and household chores. If Dad can help with the baby, and cooking and cleaning, then Mom will have more time to *share the love*. And what is sexier than a man doing dishes? The more help Mom receives, the more time she will have to feel normal again and the more desire she will have toward her spouse.

If you are finding that despite any changes made, you're still not in the mood, have a talk with your partner. You may have to reassure him that it won't be like this forever—you'll get your mojo back soon—but you need more time.

Date Nights Are Important

When was the last time you went out on a date with your spouse? Watching a movie together after the kids have gone to bed is a great idea—if you manage to stay awake. But I'm talking about hiring a babysitter, dressing up, and going out somewhere for romance and/or fun. It doesn't happen for many new parents; I know. Who has the energy (let alone the time) to go out with your significant other? A parent's busy and active lifestyle likely puts romantic date nights at the bottom of the priority list. Often, it is not even on the list. Dating is simply overlooked, but that can be remedied.

You *have* to schedule date nights when you're married with children—add that to your weekly scheduling meetings! It's crucial to maintaining a strong relationship because quality couple time is just what you need for a healthy marriage. Date nights help to rekindle the romance that is often put on the back burner when you're tending to the day-to-day bustle.

I try to arrange a night out as often as possible, firstly because I *need* to get out of the house and secondly because *we* need it as a couple. Ideally, outings should happen at least once a month, but realistically, we can fit in a night on the town only every few months.

If it's been longer than two months since your last couple's outing, then you need to change that immediately. Book a babysitter or get your mother-in-law to come over to watch the kids and go out as a couple. You both deserve a little fun!

Fun Date Ideas

- Skip the routine dinner and a movie; do something different and fun. Go bowling or skating. Find a roller-skating rink and remember what it was like to moonlight in seventh grade. If you have only a couple of hours during the weekend to get out without baby, hop on some bicycles and go for a ride together. Or throw on your running shoes and go for a long walk and a coffee at your local shop. Keep it simple and close to home so you don't have to worry about being away from baby too long—especially if you are nursing.

- If you're not the type to get active on a date (I don't mean *that* kind of active), grab your loved one and head to the bookstore. Pick up a couple of lattes and some biscotti, find a corner in the romance section, and read each other some poetry. Find a steamy romance novel or Kama Sutra book and take it home with you to read together in bed.

- Plan a romantic picnic in the middle of your living room floor. Lay out a blanket, feed your partner some cheese

Before kids · Date Night

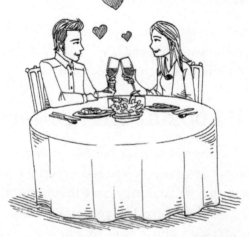

After kids

and grapes, and share a bottle of wine. Don't forget to turn on the fireplace and play some soft, sensual music . . . as long as it's not Michael Bolton.

- Married couples don't need to worry about looking cheap. Hey, having kids is expensive! Search the net for group-buying coupon companies that offer great deals on entertainment experiences. You can find yourself saving up to half price on museums, wine tastings, restaurants, and even massages—now that's a date!

You don't need much time or have to spend a lot of money to reconnect with your husband. Even just a couple of hours alone with Hubby can do wonders for your marriage.

You'll Look at Him Differently

Once you become a parent, you see your spouse in a different way. You discover a new sense of love and respect for your spouse. Of course, you will love your baby more than anything, but you will love your baby differently than your spouse. Once you see your gorgeous husband taking care of your beautiful baby, your heart will grow more for him than you thought possible. You may find yourself falling in love with your spouse all over again!

When you see your husband holding your baby, you'll fully realize you both created this beautiful human being *together*. When you're having a tough time, remind yourself that you're both learning how to be parents; just as you're having to adjust, so is he. Understanding goes a long way.

When baby starts to smile and coo, these are the moments that will bring you both closer together. There is something so special about having created a life together that bonds you in a way like no other. And now, taking care of that little life as a team will give you newfound respect and love for your guy.

He'll also take care of you, wanting to nurture you and baby. He'll hopefully be loving and caring to ensure that you are comfortable and happy, along with baby. You can't help but look at him adoringly; the way he looks at his baby and looks at you—you're the mother of his child, after all.

Dad to Mom

That's right; it's Dad turn to share a little wisdom with us. It is only fair that we give him a chance too.

Be patient with your husband, as he's learning the ropes of being a new dad. Guide him gently—he'll follow your lead and have some good ideas to contribute as well. —Genio Carbone

When a newborn enters the world, it's inevitable that your life changes, as baby becomes the number one priority in your life. More demands are put on you and, obviously, more pressure. You are mentally and physically exhausted, and your normal schedule comes to a screeching halt. In some cases, romance goes out the window: you are in a different state of mind. Communication is definitely one of the keys to staying afloat. First and foremost, make sure you sit down and ask each other honestly what each other's expectations are and evaluate if they have been met. That is the key to longevity. —Egidio Tari

Never go to bed angry at each other. Sometimes you have to look at things from his point of view. Dads have to stay involved no matter what; read all you can, and don't worry about making mistakes. We can learn from our spouses and grow to be better people. —Coste Lianos

Never underestimate the ability and resolve of the dad to be actively and enthusiastically involved. There is a certain alpha-male typecast that exists in the media . . . and honestly in some mom circles when it comes to husbands being dads. It suggests that we need to be told what to do and how to do it, when, in fact, we are often just as ready and prepared as our spouse. When we were expecting our eldest over fifteen years ago, I attended every single prenatal appointment with my wife and I was equally involved in the planning leading up to our son's birth. I know many, many other dads who were just like that, but we don't see this representation in the media.

Being a dad isn't part of who I am. It IS who I am. The nanosecond I first heard my newborn baby cry, I was hit by a virtual sledgehammer of reality. I knew at that very moment that my life going forward would no longer be about me, and it was a reality that both humbled and excited me at the same time. —Eric Novak

Mom to Mom

I think life in general changes as you experience certain milestones. For us, our relationship changed after our first in a more positive way. We were both very supportive and worked more as a team. My husband was very supportive through very difficult times after birth . . . breastfeeding, deciding to co-sleep, etc. We never really discussed prior to having kids what type of parents we would be. It just happened and all came together on its own. I'm very thankful that we parent in similar ways and see things eye to eye. I didn't know myself what kind of parents we would be. We are now closer and more in tune with not only our children but with each other. —Michelle Gemmell

Once things settle and you're getting a little more sleep and into a routine, you fall in love with your partner even more and in such a different way. . . . Seeing them interact/ protect/play with and love on this little person you created together makes your heart swell. —Tania Pollard

I think if you let parenting change your relationship, then it will—hopefully for the better. My husband and I grew together and became closer as a couple because we created life after we had love. When you are so in love with someone and you create life, there is nothing else that means more. It brings you together in a way I can't even describe.
—Ashley-Chris Isabella

We tried for seven long years of fertility and testing, and finally, after almost giving up, we got pregnant! This little miracle has made our marriage stronger every day. Of course, we suffered less sleep and less sex, but our very strong marriage feels blessed every day. Our little man recently turned four, and our marriage is just as wonderful as the moment I peed on that marvelous little stick.
—Sabrina Lang

Chapter Sixteen

OTHER RELATIONSHIPS WILL CHANGE

You already know things are bound to change with your partner after baby's arrival. But did you ever consider how having a baby changes other relationships? As with any major life transition, having a baby can affect all relationships—including those with your family and friends.

Family Relations

After the excitement of baby's arrival begins to fade and the family has settled into routines, you may begin to encounter some friction between you and your parents and in-laws. Often, there can be a sort of power struggle among family members.

Some parents instinctively strike a good balance of supporting new moms while still giving them needed space and autonomy.

Others feel that since they had a child thirty years ago, they know everything and must convince you to do things as they did. You may feel as though your mother or mother-in-law is trying to take over or get too involved. She may stick her nose into your business, mothering, and parenting skills—and even your marriage. You may feel pushed to bottle-feed, use a pacifier, go out on date nights, not go out, be a stay-at-home mom, or put your baby to sleep on her side. You may feel like they are being judgemental rather than supportive. You might feel like you have to justify every single parenting choice you make. Older relatives may be simply curious or just nosy to know every detail about your parenting choices and daily routine. Yikes!

Sometimes the comments and advice they'll dish out will not sit well with you! Here is one example and how you might react:

Relative: "When my babies were little, they'd sleep on their stomachs."

You: "Well, they don't now . . . they say it's best to lay them on their backs."

Relative: "How much is baby eating? Is baby getting enough breast milk?"

You: "Yes, he is."

Relative: "How do you know if your breasts are producing enough milk?"

You: "Well, baby is full; baby is obviously peeing by all the wet diapers."

Relative: "Why don't you let me feed the baby?"

You: "But I'm not bottle-feeding."

Relative: "But why?"

You: "The baby doesn't like the bottle. He won't drink from it. Yes, I've tried, and he just cries. So it doesn't make sense if he's with me anyway; I can easily breastfeed."

Relative: "But I WANT to feed him too."

You: "Well, you can't!"

Suddenly the introduction of baby is creating a battleground with you and your parents, in-laws, or other family members. Once you hear the comment "It's your child, but she's my grand-child!" the territorial struggle begins!

How to Deal with the Criticism

It's quite common for some initial friction with family members, especially among parents and in-laws. You may be asked a ton of questions about your parenting choices and be on the receiving end of many side-eyes and even the stinkeye from relatives about how you choose to hold, feed, change, or even treat your baby! While you want to reply with expletives, you'll have to gently say, "I am the mother. Please respect my decisions!"

In 2017, the University of Michigan in cooperation with the C. S. Mott Children's Hospital National Poll on Children's Health asked a national sample of mothers of children zero to five years old about their perceptions of being criticized about their parenting. Most mothers (61 percent) said they have been criticized about their parenting choices, most frequently by family—their spouse/the child's other parent (36 percent), their in-laws (31 percent), or their own mother or father (37 percent).[69]

If you feel you are being questioned about your parenting decisions, be calm and respond firmly and politely. Hopefully the direct response will put Grandma or Aunt Bessie in her place. If she continues to question you, just use the doctor card. "Well, his pediatrician says that . . ." Grandma or Aunt Bessie can't possibly argue with a medical professional who specializes in children's health—though they may anyway.

What a new mom would rather hear is gentle advice from her elders. We'd be more inclined to listen to Nanna say "I remember burping my baby this way. Can I show you?" rather than "When I had my kids, we knew how much they were eating because of the bottle."

Thirty years ago, things were different. Kids didn't ride in car seats; they sat on their mother's laps while dad was smoking in the car. I think I'll trust modern-day research and scientific studies rather than what Aunt Toula did in the 1970s!

Sometimes You Need to Have It Out

New grandparents must learn boundaries, and your job is to explain how boundaries will work in your home. Be assertive with whomever is causing you grief. Sometimes you need to have it out with your mom. If you can't deal with your in-laws, your husband should. If your mother-in-law is too intrusive, ask your partner to have a chat with her. He'll need to step up and speak on your behalf. You shouldn't have to be dealing with any family drama.

He can gently remind her that he realizes her good intentions and that she has gone through parenthood before but that things have changed since then. There are new ways of child-rearing and parenting that have evolved through science and research. While you appreciate her advice and guidance, remind her that this is a new experience that new Mom and Dad would like to have an opportunity to enjoy on their own. Tell her to use a gentle approach rather than spit out advice. Ask her to share advice when you or your partner ask for it. This will make mother-in-law much more approachable and likeable.

Many times, it's simply a matter of a power struggle between the two women. Everyone is becoming accustomed to their new roles, which can sometimes be blurred. Although it may seem difficult at the time, try to be empathetic—your parents and/or his are trying to figure out this dynamic as well. They're excited to be grandparents—they will want to spend time with their grandchild too. You can all find a middle ground where everyone feels respected and happy.

On the Flip Side

On the other side of the coin, you may harbor feelings of resentment that you're *not* getting the help you need. Your family is practically nonexistent now that baby is born. You only wish you had the overbearing parents! You dream of having a nagging mother to come over and sit with you and the baby or fold your laundry and make you a pot of chicken soup.

Sometimes your family members or friends feel they are bothering you, so they stay away. I have to say it—friends who don't have kids won't get it. They are secretly afraid or intimidated by this little person who has taken over your life. I had friends who never came to visit me once my baby was born. The time I needed company most, someone who could offer an ear or even a hand to hold the baby, weren't there. If this happens, there is a huge feeling of disappointment. Try not to judge; they may just not know what to do, so, sadly, they do nothing.

Somewhere in the middle is where you want to be. You want your family to be a part of your baby's life but in moderation. Drop-ins at eight in the morning on a weekend are not helpful, unless they are bringing extra-large coffees and a box of donuts. Long visits are also a big no-no, unless they are coming over to help clean, cook, and do laundry any time after eleven in the morning with a phone call ahead of time to ask if you are free.

Do your best to say "yes" when this happens, and you are likely to receive a batch of soup or a casserole!

The Good News

At some point in a woman's life, after having kids, this realization hits you smack in the face. You suddenly see yourself in the mirror and have an epiphany—*OH MY GOSH, I'm becoming my mother!*

After becoming a mom, you will have a new appreciation for your own mother. *NOW I realize what being a mother is. Now I know why I drove her crazy—all the work she did to raise us, putting up with the three of us, working full time, taking care of the house, cooking elaborate meals, entertaining relatives on the weekends, and even sewing us clothes. How did she do it all? She made it look so EASY.* You will be calling up your mom and thanking her. BECAUSE NOW YOU GET IT!

You have new respect for your dad, too! Of course, you never realize how great your parents are until you have your own children. You'll understand why they made the choices and sacrifices they did, because you are now filling those shoes.

You'll also realize that there should be no power struggle. Baby's grandparents need their own bonding time with the baby without you hovering. You'll feel like they are trying to raise your kids their way, and that puts your back up for sure. Later, you'll realize that your child has much to learn and gain from his relationship with his grandparents.

I learned new things about my own children when they spent time *alone* with their grandparents. Give your growing child an opportunity to make memories with their grandparents and create their own bond. You then realize, *These family members are helping to shape my child's identity!* Think ahead on these future moments, and keep a great relationship now when baby is brand new.

Things You May Hear from Friends and Even Strangers

If you're a new mother, you will undoubtedly hear various comments from family, friends, and even strangers. Because you're a new mother, people seem to think they have free reign to blurt out inappropriate things, ask personal questions, and dish out their own opinions and judgments—even if you didn't ask for them. Here are a few common things you may hear.

"Oh yeah; I've been there, done that."

This is not what a first-time mom wants to hear. It sounds as if the person doesn't care because they've already gone through the sleepless nights, the cluster feeding, and the explosive diapers. You can politely say, "Well, that's great, but I'm going through it NOW." Your hope is that they will empathize with you and, rather than brush off your concerns, offer real advice on how to get through the challenges.

Instead of being upset by the comment, ask "Do you remember how it was, how you felt?" Really listen if they have anything helpful to share. Perhaps they will suddenly remember how hard it was when they were in the thick of being a new parent.

Don't let anyone downplay what you're feeling just because they've gone through it themselves. You're entitled to feel the way you feel and share your thoughts on it.

"I'm sure you can't wait until your baby is old enough to do things on his own."

Wait—isn't the growing-up part one of the joys of having a child? Watching every baby develop and reach milestones is so precious. You don't want to hurry it all up just so that they can be independent. You don't want your child to crawl and walk quite yet. Enjoy it while you can!

Revel in each stage, whether they need to be held or can sit up on their own. Watch your child learn to crawl around and explore his surroundings. Sure, it'll be more challenging, as you'll need to be there every step along the way! Yes, you'll be exhausted from running after your Olympic sprinter, but when you watch your kid manage to scoot across the room at record speed, you can't help but marvel at each milestone.

"It goes by too fast! Enjoy every moment!"

You'll hear this one from the moms who haven't had a baby or toddler in a few years . . . they're already missing the early years of their child's life when they were dependent on their Mommy. But a mom who has had to change her shirt three times after having her baby projectile-vomit on her isn't going to want to enjoy each and every moment. Instead, tell us that we're doing a great job as a new mother and that we're going to be just fine!

"Oh, just you wait!"

Uh oh . . . there's nothing more fearful than being warned that things are not going to get any easier. "Just wait until the terrible twos kick in!" "Just wait until they start school and have an attitude!" "Just wait until they are a teenager!"

I realize that parenting is challenging, but it's challenging at every phase and stage. Different types of challenges, but challenges nonetheless! I don't want to be frightened by your horror stories. Instead, tell me about the fun stages too and how amazing they'll be despite the challenges, temper tantrums, and attitude. Tell me that my love for them is only going to grow stronger as their personalities form. Make me want to look forward to the future and all the fun times ahead!

"Time for another one!"

I heard this one almost immediately after my first was born. Was it a race? How quickly was I expected to have a second child?! I'd just reply with a snarky "Seriously?" That'll usually do the trick. If and when you have another child is your business.

I Didn't Ask for Your Advice

You've spent nine months receiving tons of advice and compliments. You have listened to beautiful and frightening stories, especially those labor/delivery stories that you didn't ask to hear, and then, finally, your precious baby arrives. Oh, the advice you will receive! Whether you like it or not, people will give you unsolicited advice. Although some of the advice may be helpful, some of it is questionable!

One comment I heard that was utterly ridiculous was from a fellow mother who eyeballed me for holding my baby too much. "Oh, you shouldn't pick up your baby all the time—they need to learn to be independent." At six months? Come on! Yes, I'll just let my six-month-old baby not depend on me at all—he should be able to change his own diaper too, right?

Here are some of the worst pieces of advice many moms receive in baby's first year.

Bad advice: "Tooth pain? Put Ouzo on his gums!" (Ouzo is a Greek anise-flavored liqueur. My Greek relative had no clue!)

Truth: A cold pacifier or teething ring stored in the refrigerator can help baby's sore gums. But keep an eye out to make sure she doesn't choke as she gnaws on it. If your baby has started solids, chilled fruit in a mesh bag specially designed for that purpose can provide some relief. You can also gently rub your baby's gums with a clean pinky finger.

The US Food and Drug Administration (FDA) warns that numbing gels or creams containing benzocaine shouldn't be used on children under two without guidance from a doctor. If nothing is working and your baby needs relief, check with baby's doctor.

Bad advice: "Baby can't sleep? Add some cereal to your baby's bottle!"

Truth: No, you should not be adding rice cereal to baby's bottle. Your baby needs only breast milk or formula for the first few months—that's it.

The American Academy of Pediatrics recommends breastfeeding as the sole source of nutrition for your baby for about the first six months. Offering cereal in a bottle (or even on a spoon) before babies are developmentally ready can increase the likelihood of gagging or inhaling the thickened mixture into their lungs. When baby is old enough to digest cereal, he should also be ready to eat it from a spoon.

Bad advice: "Substitute milk with juice at six months."

Truth: You shouldn't add juice to a bottle (and let your baby's teeth rot from the crazy amounts of sugar). I wouldn't give much juice to a toddler either. Keep juice to a minimum. Too much juice, especially apple juice, can cause diarrhea. Also, baby will have less appetite for nutritious food if they are drinking too much juice.

Bad advice: "You should give your baby water, not just breast milk."

Truth: Breast milk is all baby needs in the first six months. Breast milk has 88 percent water anyway!

Bad advice: "You can't get pregnant if you're breastfeeding."

Truth: Hmmm, I wonder how many women took that advice and were in for a total shock two months later! Most breastfeeding moms experience lactation amenorrhea, which means they have little or no periods at all. While they may believe they are not ovulating, becoming pregnant while breastfeeding can and does happen.

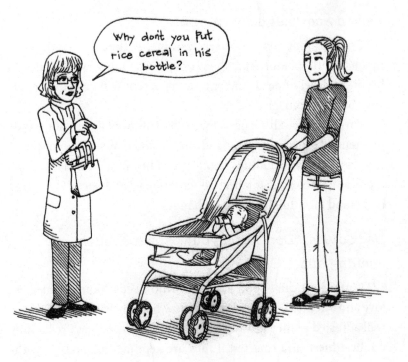

Bad advice: "Give your baby Dimetapp!"

Truth: Don't give your baby antihistamines and deconges-tants! These medicines have not been shown to be safe or effective in children younger than six years.

Bad advice: "You shouldn't sleep with your baby in the same room."

Truth: In fact, room-sharing for the first six months helps your baby sleep safely and lowers the risk of SIDS. The American Academy of Pediatrics recommends room-sharing as an ideal sleep environment.[70]

Bad advice: "Let her cry it out."

Truth: If you consider sleep training, it shouldn't even be a thought until six months at the very earliest. Only the baby knows his or her level of need, and you as the parent will be able to read your baby's language the best.

Various research suggests that babies allowed to cry alone and unattended experience panic and anxiety and may suffer long-term negative effects, including chemical and hormonal imbalances in the brain, decreased intellectual, emotional, and social development, and harmful physiologic changes.[71]

Bad advice: "Don't hold your baby too much—it's spoiling him."

Truth: You can't spoil an infant who needs Mom and Dad's love and attention. In fact, studies show holding baby makes them well adjusted as they grow. Research shows that babies are happiest, healthiest, and smartest if they are kept in close contact with their mother or another family member most of the time.

Bad advice: "Wake the baby every two to three hours to feed."

Truth: Unless baby woke on his own, I wasn't waking him up! Unless it's the first few weeks when baby is regaining weight and you're getting your milk in and settling into a schedule, there is no need to wake baby up so often. Most babies will wake up by themselves. It's also best not to wake babies at night so that they find their own schedule.

Bad advice (or, at least, questionable): "It gets easier."

Truth: Myth or truth, I don't think it ever gets any easier. Perhaps the physical part, meaning chasing your toddler around so that he doesn't hurt himself, eases. But the emotional challenges of parenthood definitely increase as kids get older. You'll never stop worrying.

The Mom Club

"Hi, I'm Maria, and this is my first baby. He's five months old and just learned to roll over. We hope to make some new friends in the area." It felt like school all over again. Trying to meet new women, hoping to build friendships, and, more importantly, finding baby buddies for my child.

The Mother Goose program was a big deal for me at that time—I was forced to put some clothes on, attempt to sleek my hair into a nice, tight ponytail rather than a raggedy bun, and put some lip gloss and deodorant on. Thankfully, the other moms were also dressed in sweatpants (this was before Lululemon was a big deal).

I was eager to interact with larger groups of other moms, and, while I was nervous, I was very excited. Shyly, I introduced myself and tried to make small talk with the other members of the group. Soon I realized that I was nodding and smiling with a big, stupid grin on my face, feeling really desperate to make new friends.

I hadn't felt so insecure about myself ever before. I felt like an extraterrestrial, with tentacles growing out of my nose and fire coming out of my mouth when I'd speak. Why was I so nervous?

I didn't realize at the time that I was feeling some anxiety along with my depression. It was time to put my big-girl panties on and take control of myself, because I am not an insecure person. I couldn't recognize that meek, insecure woman in the mirror anymore when I was such a confident person before motherhood.

I wondered if it was this hard for other parents to make friends. But it was time for me to join the Mom Club and try to mesh with the other women.

Friendships

You'll want to lean on your friends now more than ever before. If you're the first in your group to have a baby, you'll want to meet some other moms like you—stat. Join a mom-and-baby class or a new mom group where you can meet other new mothers. You'll find comfort in talking to other women who are going through similar stages and challenges. Sharing stories and tips and coming to the realization that you're not alone is so helpful.

How do you find them? Meeting new mom friends is a little like dating. We're scared to make the first move. Say the wrong thing, and you'll scare off a potential friend. Keep your cool so they think you're someone fun to hang around with. And then the hardest part—asking for their phone number.

If you're solo, the park is a great way to meet some new mom friends as well. At first, you may feel awkward trying to strike up a conversation. My first thought was *Well, these women probably already have a group of friends—they're not looking for more.* The truth is, many of these other new moms are feeling just like you—looking for another adult to talk to! I mean, baby talk can get a little tiresome after a while!

Look online for local mom meetup groups. Similar to dating apps, there are apps to meet new mom friends too. It's as easy as posting *Hey, I'm a new mom, looking for some new mom friends to go for walks and meet at the park. Message me!* I've seen this on an almost weekly basis on a local mom group I run on Facebook, and every time, there are at least a dozen responses from other moms looking for friendship too.

Even if you do meet a bunch of new mom friends, it still can be challenging to find the right one or two. You may gravitate to moms with babies around the same age as yours who can play well together! (If one baby keeps pulling the hair of another, it's probably a sign that these babies are not going to be best friends.) Their naps may need to be around the same time, too, so you can actually coordinate time to get together. It's all very complicated—but worth the effort!

What if you don't feel like part of a mom club? While many commercials and YouTube videos encourage a unity among all mothers, the real truth is many of us prefer to surround ourselves with like-minded people. If you don't find yourself fitting in to one particular group, then you may feel excluded.

Oh no—memories of elementary school are flooding back! The jocks, the geeks, the popular group, the rockers, the punks . . . and now those are replaced with the granola moms, the babywearing moms, the helicopter moms, the tiger moms, the fashionistas. These are labels we've created ourselves, as much as I dislike them. But the reality is that you will identify yourself with one of these groups more than others. You'll be drawn to certain women because they have similar values, ideas, and thoughts. Unless you don't. Then you ask yourself: *Where do I fit in?* The answer isn't always easy.

Find a supportive group of other women who will take you as you are. The last thing you need is a group of judgmental women who will question every parenting choice you make. Friends are meant to uplift and enhance—not barrage and bring down. I think all new moms are desperate to make friends and need to make a connection with someone who is going through a similar situation. Just go for it!

While relationships with your parents, in-laws, family members, and friends may change after baby is born, many of these changes will be for the good, creating a deeper bond and support for your new family. Make the effort to seek out new friends too. New moms who are right there in the trenches with you can enrich and inspire you—and don't forget to lift up and inspire that new friend right back. We all need each other!

Chapter Seventeen

YOUR BODY WILL CHANGE

We have one life. I don't want to spend my time thinking about the size of my arse. I want to be as healthy as I can be, and I want to have as much fun as I can have. I want to be around for my children. That's it. Those are the priorities. Not getting a flat stomach.

—Kate Winslet

have stretch marks, and I wear a bikini. I have a somewhat flabby middle, and I wear a bikini. I also have cellulite, and I wear a bikini. My boobs sag, but I wear a bikini with support.

I wear that bikini because I earned the right! My body carried two babies for nine months each. My ever-changing body was a vessel to two lives. I wear my bikini because I know what my body is capable of, and it's freaking amazing. Those C-section scars or stretch marks or saggy skin aren't scars—they are tiger stripes.

No one can fully prepare you for the changes your body undergoes during pregnancy, childbirth, and even after baby arrives. Once the baby is out, the focus is on caring for the child. But mama will need to take some time to work on herself too.

Blog: Gone South

Wednesday, July 9, 2008

Having a baby means that your body has changed and, for most of us, will never be quite the same again . . . unless you're Heidi Klum. (Does that woman have any stretch marks? Perhaps that million-dollar camera and airbrushing computer has something to do with that phenomenon.) If you're like me, you tried sweating those last ten pounds off at home by buying an elliptical machine and a bunch of Tae Bo DVDs. Yoga just won't cut it.

Now the elliptical is gathering dust, the P90X DVD is warped, and you've managed to gain another five pounds. You blame it on breastfeeding—your body needs that extra fat to help produce milk. But your belly hangs over your jeans, your stretch marks are starting to turn silver, and you don't know if you'll ever get back into those pre-pregnancy jeans. Perhaps it's time for a little bonfire.

So now what? Call Jenny Craig? After months of deliberation, I joined a gym. After just a few workouts, my body awoke from hibernation. My butt started to tighten again, and I could catch a glimpse of my long-lost abdominal muscles that I thought had gone away for good. Yeah! Excitement! I could get that twenty-something body back!

Oh, but wait . . . two kids later, who am I kidding? No matter how many minutes I do on the treadmill and how many weights I can lift, am I still going to have a flabby belly and loose skin? Let's not forget the boobs . . . those perky girls I enjoyed in my twenties have now gone south.

Even worse, my boobs were small before, and after breastfeeding two hungry boys, they're even smaller now! They have deflated permanently. I've done the test; place a pencil under your breasts and see if they hold it up; if it stays, they sag. For me, that pencil is pretty well secured! Heck, I could store a piece of gum under there, my keys, my wallet . . .

A boob lift and a tummy tuck sound so tempting! Whether I could actually go through with a surgical procedure is another story. After watching shows like Dr. 90210, I'm not so sure. I've seen how they stuff those huge silicone implants into that tiny little hole where your nipple should be but has been cut out temporarily during the surgery—yikes! Looks like I'm going to have to learn to deal with my girls as they are—perhaps imperfect but at least intact.

Body Changes after Children

The truth is, your body will likely never return to its previous state after giving birth. The taut muscles you flaunted as a teen have now loosened to allow baby to grow. The tight skin on the back of your thighs is now covered in dimples—and not the cute ones. The cute belly button is now stretched sideways instead of that magazine-perfect vertical oval and covered in silver markings.

These, my dear readers, are not what you think—no, they are more than stretch marks and cellulite—they are battle scars of a forever-changing you. They are permanent reminders of the beautiful creature you've miraculously created.

I have my moments where I'll look at my body with a side-eye. But as I look closer, I lay my finger upon the grooves of those markings . . . and celebrate the wonder and joy of bringing a child into this world. Through my growing womb and painful labor, I became a mother—a nurturer and care provider to my offspring.

Aside from the beautiful outcome, let's get real about what happens to your body.

Stretch Marks

Stretch marks are more common than you think—they occur in 50 to 90 percent of women. These marks are caused both by the skin stretching and by the effects of hormonal changes on fibers in the skin. They begin as red or purple stripes as your skin grows, fading to pale or flesh-color after pregnancy that will generally be permanent. Yahoo.

I was lucky with my first baby; I didn't experience many stretch marks on my belly even though I gained weight rapidly. I made sure to keep my skin moisturized. Maybe I should thank my parents for their genes.

But that all went out the window with my second . . . I gained weight steadily with my second pregnancy, moisturized, ate well, etc. But within a few weeks, his growth skyrocketed, and the skin on my belly couldn't keep up.

The fun part is that stretch marks don't tan, so if you think laying out in the sun will help diminish their appearance, they'll only stand out more. Sunscreen is your friend here, ladies. You can also continue to moisturize after baby is born—it can't hurt, but don't expect lotions or scar creams to remove your stretch marks. You are going to have to make peace with your skin.

Abdominal Separation

During pregnancy, about one-third of women experience a separation of their stomach muscles known as diastasis recti. During pregnancy, the growth of the fetus exerts pressure on abdominal cavity muscles, in particular the rectus abdominis. When there is rapid growth or weaker abs, the pressure can cause the rectus abdominis muscle to separate along the linea alba, creating a split between the left and right sides.

The muscle can separate! Imagine that your belly is pushing everything upward and outward. Those little feet in the womb are doing some amazing work. The good news is, many cases of diastasis recti correct themselves after birth, but some do not—in those cases, exercise can help and sometimes surgery is needed.

Saggy Belly Skin

Your tummy may also not be the same again. While you may have a C-section scar to deal with, you'll also have some extra storage in your belly and a little extra skin too. Your tummy may look like a wrinkled old map for a while!

Remember—it takes six weeks for your uterus to go back to its original size. Don't assume that your belly will be completely flat after six weeks; it will take longer for most women.

But that extra cushion was a haven for my baby—it became his lovey. Any time he wanted comfort, his hand was right there touching and caressing my belly. He'd plant his little cherub face right into my tummy, kissing it, giving it raspberries. How easily you can forget about that extra weight and skin with moments like those.

Saggy Breasts

Your breasts will be full and engorged while you're breastfeeding . . . you'll enjoy the 2x cup size. But when you stop nursing? Wa wa waaaaa.

Your breasts grow and deflate as the milk comes and goes . . . but when the milk is done, those boobies are going to deflate permanently. You will miss the engorgement and extra cleavage if you're already small-chested. You may look in the mirror and think, *Gee, my breasts look kind of sad.*

As soon as the milk supply stops, regardless of whether you breastfeed or not, the ligaments are left looser and further stretched out, causing the breasts to shrink and sag. Invest in a good push-up bra!

YOUR BODY WILL CHANGE

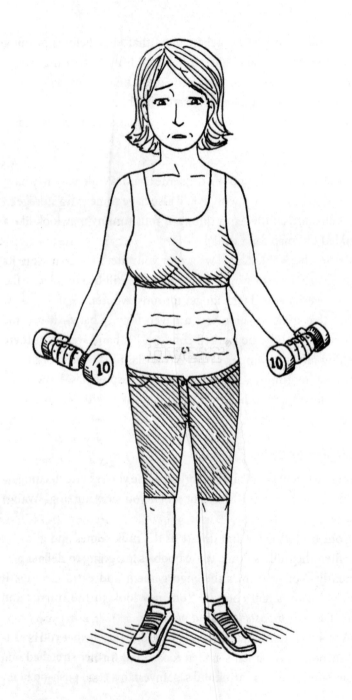

I'm telling you, you'll mourn a little bit when the breastfeeding ends. These knockers provided sole nourishment for the first six months. How cool is that!

Your Hips May Stay Wider

During the third trimester, pregnancy hormones cause the ligaments holding the pelvic girdle together to soften, which allows the birth canal to widen during labor and delivery.

After giving birth, diet and exercise can take care of the extra weight your body is carrying. As for the looser ligaments, they will firm up over time, but your pelvis may never return to its exact pre-pregnancy shape. Hey—a baby just traveled through there, so your pants may be up a size permanently.

But you have curves now! Your waist-to-hip ratio is more proportioned, voluptuous . . . bright side.

Your Feet May Stay Bigger

My feet went from a size nine to a size ten. Once my baby was born, I looked at my closet and thought, *I'm never going to be able to fit back into my shoes again: my strappy heels and knee-high riding boots!* I felt like the bones in my feet had stretched out sideways. Would they go back to their previous size? Apparently not.

I tried squeezing my chubby toes back into my stiletto heels, but my scrunched-up toes couldn't take the pain. At that point, I figured I may as well wear flip-flops since none of my shoes fit (and I wasn't about to buy a bunch of new shoes and boots). I thought maybe if I dropped some weight, I could salvage my footwear.

Teeth

This one was a big shocker to me, and it may be to you as well. Your teeth may never be the same again. *Come again?!* Pregnancy can lead to dental problems in some women, including gum disease and increased risk of tooth decay. During pregnancy, your increased hormones can affect your body's response to plaque (the layer of germs on your teeth).

I feel like my babies sucked every vitamin and mineral out of my body, including calcium and vitamin D. My near-perfect oral health turned into cavities and gum disease after children. While I'd like to place all the blame on my kids, I think aging affects dental issues as well as being too darn exhausted after childbirth to have proper dental care. (Raise your hand if you've been too tired to brush your teeth before bed!) An electric toothbrush does all the work for you; even half-asleep, you can manage to hold the spinning brush up to your mouth. And the cost of that magical, energy-saving toothbrush is well worth the money saved on fillings!

Your Thick, Gorgeous Hair Will Now Fall Out

The thick locks you so enjoyed as a pregnant woman will soon start to shed.

When pregnant, hormones made your hair stay on your head rather than flow down the shower drain, which is why your hair seemed thicker. But after you've given birth and your hormones have settled down, the hair goes into a shedding phase. Like a dog, really. About three months after delivery, the hair will start to come out, seemingly, by the fistful.

On a normal day, you lose about one hundred hairs, but that number skyrockets during this time to about five hundred a day. Don't worry; you're not losing all of your hair! Just don't be alarmed when you find handfuls of hair coming out.

After a few more months, your hair should be back to the way it was pre-pregnancy, but you may not have the same hair as you did before. Some women have a change in texture: more curls, less curls, more wiry, or less body. And whether age plays a part is only your business, but you may see a few more gray hairs—though I prefer to think of these as highlights.

You Will Leak

Did you ever think that along with the stretch marks, leaky breasts, and extra weight, you'd have to also deal with a weak bladder? Well, sheesh, after all that pushing, even if you've had a C-section, muscles in that entire area take a beating.

You can cough or sneeze, even laugh hysterically, and suddenly, pee is running down your leg. You'll run to the bathroom, but you just don't make it in time. Now you need to make a quick change of panties. And did you wonder why your mom never jumped on the trampoline? Well, now you get it; it is better to not add pressure down there. Especially in the first few months after childbirth.

Bladder incontinence, or light bladder leakage, is one of the most common problems experienced by new moms, affecting about a third in the first year after having their baby. So if you're experiencing this, you are not alone!

It takes time for those pelvic muscles to heal after giving birth. Do those Kegels, ladies, and tighten those bits!

I wasn't in a race [to lose the baby weight]. I was really kind to myself because I was actually really impressed with the fact that I had just had a baby, like "I made a human!" —Pink

Blog: Dribble

March 30, 2008
Ever feel like your life is so hectic you can't catch your breath? Sometimes I forget to even pee, and I end up running to the bathroom just in time before my bladder explodes.

Yes, I have wet my pants running to the toilet. And sometimes I'm in such a rush to pee that I'll plop down on the toilet, not realizing that the toilet seat has been left up, and almost fall right in.

For some, this is what happens after having kids—no bladder control. I'll cough or sneeze and I'll leak. Or dribble. Requiring a change of underwear. Ugh. Luckily it's only happened at home so far, but there will be the day when I'm out and get completely embarrassed. Pantiliners save lives.

I never thought I'd have bladder incontinence at my age! The thought of wearing Depends in my thirties frightens me. Add that to my growing list of older-age products that I'm already starting to use (including gray-resistant hair dyes, control-top panties, and girdle-type garments), and I'm depressed just thinking about it.

I remember while pregnant my doctor told me to do Kegels because conditioned muscles make birth easier and your perineum will more likely be intact—meaning fewer tears and episiotomies. I did them religiously. Anything to make labor easier. But I still tore. Only the doctor and God know how many stitches I got. Sitting on an ice pack for three days and taking two months to heal is not a result of just a few.

Don't you love when the books tell you to massage your perineum? Imagine yourself: your pregnant belly is out to there, your legs are swollen, you now officially have "cankles." You're lying on the couch, watching reruns of "Family Ties"—and you're spread eagle, massaging the area between your vagina and your derriere! Lovely! All that work and preparation . . . isn't it enough that we have to prepare ourselves mentally and physically for labor—now we have to prepare our freaking vaginas too?

It obviously didn't work for me! So what's a girl to do? Gotta do those Kegels! Three sets three times a day—and no one will even notice. Just try not to go cross eyed in the line at Target while you squeeze and hold, two, three, four . . . yes, you can do them anytime, anyplace . . . it's your little secret . . . I could be doing them

*right now as I'm writing this! You're reading and already did your
set—nice work!!*

Losing the Weight

Gisele Bündchen rocked a bikini just six months after giving birth
to her baby boy, Benjamin. The supermodel has amazing genes,
obviously, but she also credits an active lifestyle during pregnancy
for her post-baby weight loss: "I did kung fu up until two weeks
before Benjamin was born and yoga three days a week."

HUH? I couldn't touch my toes by the eighth month, let alone
jump around doing kung fu moves!

If you're one of those women who can exercise up until birth,
kudos to you. I was pretty much waddling like a penguin by the
seventh month of pregnancy. No matter how healthy I ate and
how active I was, the weight kept packing on. It was like a soft,
protective padding that was beyond my control.

Don't compare yourself to a celebrity who has access to personal trainers, chefs, and nannies and whose job is to look good.
Most of us moms are regular people who do our best day in and
day out. That is the true perfect!

But is the pressure on women to lose the weight quickly, as
quickly as celebrity moms? Seeing media images of women fitting back into their pre-pregnancy jeans within three months has
a subconscious effect on some. But why add that kind of pressure
to yourself? There is no rush. The weight will take time to come
off. Nine months to put the weight on, nine months to take it off!
Some of us would like to fit back into our jeans so we don't have to
buy a new wardrobe. Stretchy pants and a little patience work just
fine—the most important thing is taking care of baby!

The Good News

There is hope. My body went back to normal about two years after my second child was born. My feet went back to normal size. I lost the weight, and most of it—except for the last twenty pounds—came off easily. The last ten were the toughest. I made a realistic weight goal for myself. I wasn't going to go back to my pre-pregnancy body or weight; it was okay to be a little heavier at thirty-something than I was in my late twenties.

It takes time and hard work to get back to normal again. And normal does not mean looking or feeling exactly as you did before baby. You may feel more feminine with your new figure and more comfortable in your own skin. Accept and embrace that new womanly, curvy body. Hips and a booty are sexy!

Mom to Mom

Do not run, laugh, or sneeze if you have to pee! —Jacqueline Robinson

Well, they make you wait six weeks until you're allowed to start an exercise program, but nobody warns you that you're gonna pee when you do jumping jacks! Just trying to tone up and get rid of mommy tummy not knowing a diaper is required. Not to mention boob sag—I was left nice and perky with my first child, but my second has robbed me of my perky, plump boobies. Life goes on. —Stefanie Puiras

Permanent mom pouch. And I didn't think my feet grew until I slowly realized none of my old shoes felt comfortable anymore. And my once-nice breasts are now sad and limp, but bigger than before. I'm a mess. —Rebeccah Beaulieu

My body became rounder. I wasn't fat, but my belly, hips, even the circumference of my chest was rounded. I am heavier now that I've had four babies, but I love it. I'm a softer body shape. I like my roundness. —Jenny DiPietro

I needed a new wardrobe after the change in where weight sits now. It also took a full year before I could sit on a wooden chair without so much pain on my tailbone. A bizarre bonus is that my eyesight improved. My doctor said I am not the only one to have that great side effect. —Monica Bertenshaw

Chapter Eighteen

YOU WILL NEVER BE THE SAME

Making the decision to have a child—it is momentous. It is to decide forever to have your heart go walking around outside your body.

—Elizabeth Stone

Being a mom changes every part of your being. You look at the world differently now that you have a child that is part of it. Your priorities shift; more than anything else, you want to protect the child you love unconditionally, you put your child's needs first, and your goals change.

The physical wounds of childbirth and pregnancy will heal, but becoming a mother will change you forever, leaving a permanent mark on your heart and soul. You'll see the world in different eyes; you'll feel more concerned, joyful, frantic, and grateful. You will care more about the world that your children will grow up in.

You'll Be a Better Person

It's cliché to say that everything changes. But it does. You may not have cared at all before about your religious upbringing, until the time comes to decide whether you will baptize your baby or not. Should your child go to Sunday school or learn their grandparents' language?

Even if you're not hugely religious yourself, do you expose your child to religion anyway? You are making important decisions for this person who will grow up with experiences that you've chosen to help shape him. This is a huge responsibility!

You will want to learn new things so you can share your new-found knowledge with your child—which also may save you when your child asks the one million questions that will soon come your way. You may never have wanted to play baseball, but, suddenly, you're finding yourself throwing a ball around and buying tickets to the next Blue Jays game.

You want to be the parent that your child will be proud of, so you will make every effort to be a better person. You want to teach your kids to love and respect others and to stand up for what's right. So you are more deliberate in the way you treat and interact with others; after all, you're now setting the example for your child.

You Become Selfless

Becoming a mother forces you to throw your needs out the window—for a little while, anyway. While you're caring for your baby those first important few months, you will have little time for yourself. But that will soon ease, and you will have time again to focus on your own health and well-being. Life will revolve around your baby, and, of course, you will do anything for her. For the first time, life isn't about you—it's about your child first.

You Love More

Having a kid is life altering, but mostly it's fantastic to love that tiny little human more than anything. You will feel proud as you become more responsible and step up to new challenges without hesitation.

The bond between parent and child is likely the strongest connection you'll ever experience. The love you feel for your baby is part of human nature; science shows parents are hardwired to love their babies. Even if you're a little nervous about parenthood, or think *How can I love this little person I haven't even met?*, biology is on your side; the explosion of love you feel will be unlike anything else.

Before having children, you don't realize just how much you could love somebody. Of course you love your spouse. But loving a child is a different kind of love. Your life before you had your child doesn't quite seem as fulfilling as it does now. You want to provide for your child, love him, protect him, and guide him the best way you can.

Your child will open your eyes up again to life's joys and force you to see the world through her sense of wonder. You'll gain a renewed sense of what your own childhood might have been like before you started having memories. You'll be filled with amazement when teaching and watching a little brain learn and develop.

You'll feel a love that you never even knew you had. There aren't any words to describe what you feel when your little one looks up at you and shows you that gummy grin or when they open their eyes wide in amusement and laugh for the first time. Nothing else seems to matter. It's the best feeling in the world.

Your Baby Loves You

You have already fallen in love with your baby, and he is falling in love with you too. From the time baby is born, he is memorizing your face and already knows your scent. When you hold him in your arms and talk to him, he recognizes your voice. Because you feed him when he's hungry, baby has learned he can trust you. Sometimes he'll quiet down as soon as he can tell he's about to eat; he knows you are taking care of him. Because you comfort him when he's upset and pick him up when he cries, he knows he can relax when you're holding him. As he gets older, he'll miss you when you leave the room and reach out for you when he sees you.

That remarkable connection goes back to the womb! It even is connected by hormones—you still get a rush of oxytocin when you see your nine-month-old baby.

What I wasn't prepared for is how much baby loves Mommy. Baby needs you more than anyone else. Yes, your partner loves you, but your children will adore you. To be surrounded by so much love warms every cell in your body. Your child gives you a renewed sense of life and a reason to get up in the morning. Your life matters more now that your baby depends on you; you have a new and important purpose as you do your best to love and teach and provide as a mother.

Deep Love through Tough Times

When you're experiencing rough times, whether in your personal or professional life, you can take one look at baby's face and know you will make it through. You HAVE to push through for her. This little life depends on you, and that feeling of unconditional love will overwhelm you. The hardships and struggles, the worries and disappointments—they all disappear when you're holding your baby in your arms.

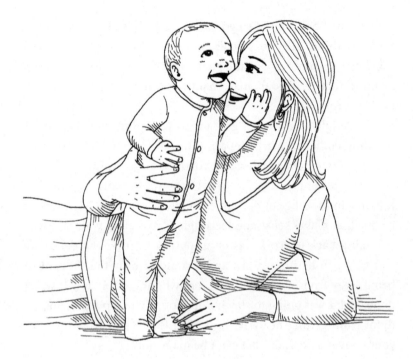

There will be times when your baby is the one having a rough day: illness, teething, and insecurities will bring you closer together as your heart goes out to that little person. Love grows as we serve others, and Mommy serving a little one—cuddling when baby is scared or not feeling well—brings you closer. Your priority is to comfort baby and make baby feel safe and loved.

Your Goals May Change

You'll tend to think of your baby first before making any decisions or taking risks. You may have spent your adult years building a career only to have it put on the back burner when you become a mother. Your desires and goals may change; while one woman may ditch the law firm to stay home and raise her family, another woman may be inspired to go back to school and earn a degree. So many things affect our goals, and certainly that new baby will spark some new decisions and goals. That's a good thing! Just keep in mind that your goals may change as you experience motherhood in real time.

You might think you'll go back to work, but then as soon as the time comes to start preparing to return, you can't bear the thought. Or you may realize that you thrive in a professional environment, leading you to find ways to continue working, whether full time in the office or part time from home. The decision should be one that makes sense and feels right for you and your family.

Going back to work wasn't an option for me. The commute was going to be impossible, and I couldn't bear the thought of being away from my baby for so many hours in the day. It was a done deal; I was going to stay home. You can't stop a determined mom from getting her way. Leaving a job to stay at home with your baby is a decision that can't be made lightly.

It is humbling not to have that second income and to need to make careful spending choices because you are on a strict household budget. It's amazing how thrifty you can become when you have to. Humility is a good thing; we quickly learned the difference between needs and wants and managed just fine with only the necessities.

There was no way I would miss out on the early months of my child's life, and I knew I would never be able to get that time back.

You May Have Less Stuff

You may decide to stay home with your baby, which means you may trade in your stilettos for Birkenstocks, your designer handbag for a canvas diaper bag, and a luxury sedan for a minivan. The carefully manicured nails and stylish pantsuit will be replaced with yoga pants and a baggy top. You will also find that baby stuff takes up space. Your antique dining table may need to make way for baby's swing and bouncy chair.

You may live more frugally, making smarter choices about how you spend your money, and even start cutting coupons. You'll be more cautious of your spending; after all, you'll have to start saving for the college fund! You'll find you will buy more for your children than for yourself, but you don't mind, because you'd rather drop all of your savings on providing the best you possibly can for your baby.

Your Schedule Will Need to Be More Flexible

Remember the times when you ran into someone you knew walking down the street and decided to grab a coffee spontaneously? (I don't either.) Being a new mom makes it challenging to drop everything on a moment's notice. You will begin to plan and schedule your life, because it takes longer to get ready and out of the house. Your schedule may also be dictated by baby for a little while; it might feel like baby is your new, rather unpredictable, personal manager!

You Will Be More Intuitive

If you didn't feel you had good intuition before having kids, you will now. You will find yourself listening more to your instincts and following your gut feelings. You will become empowered by the *knowing* of things . . . as soon as you begin to trust your instincts and get used to being a mom, you will feel empowered.

Your mission is to keep your child safe and protected. You'll realize when your baby's cry is not a regular cry or when he needs to be seen by the doctor. You'd never think you were capable of doing a flip backward to catch your baby as he began to fall off the chair, but you managed to catch him. Those Mama Bear instincts will be in full force.

While I co-slept with my baby, I was stirred instinctively when he started to rouse. You always seem to be one step ahead of baby, grabbing the nursing pillow just before he's about to wail. It doesn't end after the first year, either. My boys are older now, and they sometimes believe it when I say I have X-ray vision.

"Mom, do you have eyes at the back of your head?"

"Yes, boys. I SEE EVERYTHING."

You will also have super hearing abilities.

Husband: "And then, what happened was . . ."

Wife: "Shhhhh. I think I hear the baby."

Silence.

Baby starts to cry.

These are the Supermom characteristics that you're proud to earn and willing to keep.

You'll Be Healthier

Having a baby makes you want to be healthy. Thoughts of your mortality will move you to want to be healthy and live a long life so you can watch your baby grow up and have kids of his own. You want to eat well, exercise, and reduce your stress so you can be around for your child. Having a baby will make you want to be a better you.

You'll Become More Empathetic

Your empathy for *all* children will pull your heartstrings. When I read about a child being hurt or ill, whether in the newspaper, on television, or on the internet, I am gutted. I run to hug my babies, cling to them, and never want to let them go. Before having children, seeing horrific things in the news didn't have such a direct impact on my emotions, but now there are times it keeps me up at night.

You'll Be More Patient

Motherhood teaches you to be considerably more patient. You have no choice but to be patient as you button all 2,459 buttons of his sleeper! It forces you to accept a different pace. As you sit back and feed your baby, you will learn how to slow down and let things take their course. You can't just tell her to eat faster—you have to learn patience.

You'll Experience More Joy

If you've forgotten how sweet life can be, your child will remind you constantly. As you watch her grow, you will see innocence in her eyes. You'll experience the exhilaration of seeing your child learn to walk, talk, run, ride a bike, taste ice cream, touch a furry animal, go on a swing, and, eventually, ride a roller coaster.

You'll Be More Mindful

You will learn to embrace the day-to-day activities that make life so sweet. You will get lost in simply watching your baby. You could literally spend hours just holding him and studying every inch of him. As you slow down and spend time on walks, you'll notice things in nature that you didn't see on your morning jog or commute. Being able to enjoy the little moments throughout the day is the key to happiness.

You Will Learn to Enjoy Each Age and Stage

As you experience each phase and stage in your child's first year, you will think, *Wow, this is the best stage ever!* And then comes the next phase, and you're left speechless again. Every moment, every memory you make seems better than the last.

When I look back to that first year, I think, *I wish I could relive those moments. I wish I knew then what I know now.* I would've slowed down, napped more, and worried less! The key to fully enjoying every stage and phase is to really acknowledge and be aware of those moments. Don't be in a hurry to watch them grow.

I've heard many moms say, "I can't wait for . . ." as if they are rushing their kids to grow up. The entire journey of motherhood is such an amazing blessing, one that we often take for granted when we're cranky, haven't slept, or are covered in vomit and snot.

When they're babies, we say, "I can't wait until they're walking."

When they're walking, we say, "I can't wait until they're talking."

When they're talking, it's "I can't wait until they start school."

Next thing you know, they'll be in grade twelve, asking for car keys and being embarrassed to be seen hugging you in public. Enjoy the journey, not only the destination, because everything changes and there is always something new just around the corner.

What I've Learned During My Mom Journey

Since becoming a mom, I've learned a thing or two:

- I've learned that I love learning new things.
- I've learned that I'll never stop learning.
- I've learned that the wisdom of elders is priceless.
- I've learned children are amazing teachers, too.

- I've learned that true friends are really hard to come by.
- I've learned that how we each view the world is really all about perception.
- I've learned to read people.
- I've learned to trust my instincts.
- I've learned not to assume anything.
- I've learned to give people the benefit of the doubt.
- I've learned to be more understanding of people.
- I've learned not to take things so personally.
- I've learned that hearing doesn't mean listening—and some people have a hard time doing either.
- I've learned that to truly live in the moment is an art.
- I've learned that reality bites but daydreaming is a great place to be.
- I've learned that you can't judge a person unless you've walked a thousand miles in their shoes.
- I've learned that relationships take a lot of effort but are worth it.
- I've learned to get by on one salary and live simply.
- I've learned to not be envious of others' material possessions.
- I've learned to enjoy the simple things in life, like morning coffee and my children's laughter.
- I've learned to take time for myself to recharge and find peace.
- I've learned not to wait for things to happen but to go after what I want.
- I've learned that no matter how old you get, you can still be young at heart.
- I've learned that no matter how many children you have, you have enough love in your heart for each child.
- I've learned to be grateful for my amazing siblings and take pride in the fact that we are close and that our children will be too.

- I've learned that some sacrifices are definitely worth making.
- I've learned mothers truly are the glue that holds a family together.
- I've learned that money makes the world go around—but it doesn't feed the soul.
- I've learned that you must pursue what you love, even if you don't get paid for it.
- I've learned that it's impossible to have it all, all at once.
- I've learned that raising children is the most rewarding yet most challenging experience of all.
- I've learned that the truly fun part of life is the journey itself.

Mom to Mom

When you become a mother, the well-being of your children is always on your mind. There is never a moment when you are not aware of where they are and how they are doing. You feel everything they feel. It's the most amazing kind of love that only mothers understand. —Heidi Hoile

I became less selfish, less vain, more patient, more protective, more vocal, more assertive. Most of all, more appreciative of my own parents. —Lauren Tobin

Motherhood has made me empathetic to each person's perspective. It's given me patience I didn't know I possessed. It's given me strength and fulfillment. —Emily Dimmell

Motherhood makes me aware each and every day of all the things I thought I knew about myself and life. Even though I was an accomplished, confident woman, parenting was the one thing that I felt I didn't have a roadmap for. It is the one thing in my life that made me second-guess every decision that I made. —Bonnie Teitelbaum Wisener

Motherhood has made me realize my true inner strength. Strength of love, strength of perseverance, and strength of loyalty. —Laurie Brander

My daughter is my world. Her needs and wants come before mine. Every day with her is precious. She has taught me how to be completely selfless. —Tara Dean Tomasic

Motherhood has made me vulnerable to every emotion and every perspective. It's given me anxiety and encouragement. It has made me less trusting, more trusting, more forgiving, fearful, confident, joyful, excited, patient, impatient, hopeful; but most of all, I have felt true undeniable love . . . it definitely opens your heart to so many things you never thought possible. —Manila Goncalves

NOTES

1. Blythe, Andrew, and Jessica Buchan, eds. *Essential Primary Care*. Chichester, West Sussex, UK: John Wiley & Sons, Inc., 2016. P. 135.

2. Yetman, Robert J., and Mark D. Hormann. *Pediatrics: PreTest Self-Assessment and Review, 14th Edition*. New York: McGraw-Hill Education, 2016. P. 82.

3. American Academy of Pediatrics, Steven P. Shelov, ed., and Tanya Remer Altmann, ed. *Caring for Your Baby and Young Child: Birth to Age 5*, 5th Edition. New York: Bantam Books, 2009. P. 121.

4. Leach, Penelope. *Your Baby & Child: From Birth to Age Five*. New York: Alfred A. Knopf, 2010. P. 108.

5. Crenshaw, Jeannette. "Care Practice #6: No Separation of Mother and Baby, With Unlimited Opportunities for Breastfeeding." *The Journal of Perinatal Education* 16, no. 3 (Summer 2007): 39–43. Accessed July 13, 2017. https://www.ncbi.nlm.nih.gov/pmc/articles/PMC1948089/.

6. "The Importance of Skin to Skin Contact." International Breastfeeding Centre, 2009. Accessed July 14, 2017. http://ibconline.ca/information-sheets/the-importance-of-skin-to-skin-contact/.

7. Mohrbacher, Nancy, and Kathleen Kendall-Tackett. *Breastfeeding Made Simple: Seven Natural Laws for Nursing Mothers*, Second Edition. Oakland, CA: New Harbinger, 2010. P. 141.

8. "A Guide to Pumping Your Milk." La Leche League International, May 2009. http://lllmarivt.org/wp-content/uploads/2012/07/Guide-to-pumping-your-milk1.pdf.

9. "Is My Baby Getting Enough Milk?" La Leche League International, from *New Beginnings* 25, no. 5 (2008): 44–45. http://www.llli.org/nb/nbsepocto8p44.html.

10. Fomon, Samuel J. "Infant Feeding in the 20th Century: Formula and Beikost." *The Journal of Nutrition* 131, no. 2 (February 2001): 409S–420S. http://jn.nutrition.org/content/131/2/409S.full.

11. Andrisani, Giovanni, and Giorgia Andrisani. "Pacifier Use May Decrease the Risk of SIDS." *Journal of Neurology and Neuroscience* 8, no. 1:120 (February 2017): ISSN 2171–6625. http://www.jneuro.com/neurology-neuroscience/pacifier-use-may-decrease-the-risk-of-sids.php?aid=18523.

12. Leach, *Your Baby & Child*. P. 64.

13. Ibid, pp. 63–64.

14. Eidelman, Arthur I., Richard J. Schanler, and the American Academy of Pediatrics. "Breastfeeding and the Use of Human Milk." *Pediatrics* 129, no. 3 (March 2012): e827–41. Accessed August 7, 2017. P. e829. http://pediatrics.aappublications.org/content/pediatrics/129/3/e827.full.pdf.

15. Ibid., p. e829–31.

16. Ibid., p. e832.

17. "Nutrition during Breastfeeding." American Pregnancy Association, May 16, 2017. Accessed June 28, 2017. http://americanpregnancy.org/breastfeeding/nutrition-during-breastfeeding/.

18. Eidelman and Schanler, "Breastfeeding and the Use of Human Milk," p. e833.

19. "Diet for a Healthy Breastfeeding Mom." BabyCenter Canada Medical Advisory Board. https://www.babycenter.ca/a3565/diet-for-a-healthy-breastfeeding-mom.

20. "Vitamin D during Pregnancy and Breastfeeding." Vitamin D Council. Accessed August 4, 2017. https://www.vitamindcouncil.org/vitamin-d-during-pregnancy-and-breastfeeding/.

21. Sachs, Hari Cheryl. "The Transfer of Drugs and Therapeutics into Human Breast Milk: An Update on Selected Topics." *Pediatrics* 132, no. 3 (September 2013): e796–e809. Accessed August 7, 2017. P. e803. http://pediatrics.aappublications.org/content/132/3/e796.

22. "Fish and Omega-3 Fatty Acids." American Heart Association. Accessed August 4, 2017. http://www.heart.org/HEARTORG/HealthyLiving/HealthyEating/HealthyDietGoals/Fish-and-Omega-3-Fatty-Acids_UCM_303248_Article.jsp#.

23. Harvard T. H. Chang School of Public Health. "Omega-3 Fatty Acids: An Essential Contribution." *The Nutrition Source*, May 26, 2015. Accessed August 4, 2017. https://www.hsph.harvard.edu/nutritionsource/omega-3-fats/.

24. Langley-Evans, Simon. *Nutrition, Health and Disease: A Lifespan Approach*, Second Edition. West Sussex, UK: Wiley Blackwell, 2015. P. 128.

25. Jacobson, Hilary. *Mother Food: A Breastfeeding Diet Guide with Lactogenic Foods and Herbs*. Rosalind Press, 2007. P. 126.

26. Ibid.

27. Mennella, Julie A. "Ontogeny of Taste Preferences: Basic Biology and Implications for Health." *The American Journal of Clinical Nutrition* 99, no. 3 (March 2014): 704S–711S. Accessed June 28, 2017. P. 706S–7S. http://ajcn.nutrition.org/content/99/3/704S.full.pdf+html.

28. Togias, Alkis, et al. "Addendum Guidelines for the Prevention of Peanut Allergy in the United States: Report of the National Institute of Allergy and Infectious Diseases–Sponsored Expert Panel." *Journal of Allergy and Clinical Immunology* 139, no. 1 (January 2017): 29–44. P. 32. http://www.jacionline.org/article/S0091-6749%2816%2931222-2/pdf.

29. "Alcohol & Breast Milk." HealthyChildren.org via the American Academy of Pediatrics. Last updated November 21, 2015. Accessed August 4, 2017. https://www.healthychildren.org/English/ages-stages/baby/breastfeeding/Pages/Alcohol-Breast-Milk.aspx.

30. "Our Mission." The Fed Is Best Foundation, 2016. https://fedisbest.org.

31. Del Castillo-Hegyi, Christie. "Letter to Doctors and Parents about the Dangers of Insufficient Exclusive Breastfeeding." The Fed Is Best Foundation, April 18, 2015. https://fedisbest.org/2015/04/letter-to-doctors-and-parents-about-the-dangers-of-insufficient-exclusive-breastfeeding/.

32. Dewey Kathryn G., Laurie A. Nommsen-Rivers, M. Jane Heinig, and Roberta J. Cohen. "Risk Factors for Suboptimal Infant Breastfeeding Behavior, Delayed Onset of Lactation, and Excess Neonatal Weight Loss." *Pediatrics* 112, no. 3 (September 2003): 607–19. http://pediatrics.aappublications.org/content/112/3/607.short.

33. Li, Ruowei, Sara B. Fein, Jian Chen, and Laurence M. Grummer-Strawn. "Why Mothers Stop Breastfeeding: Mothers' Self-Reported Reasons for Stopping During the First Year." *Pediatrics* 122, Suppl. 2 (October 2008): S69–76. Pp. S73–4. http://pediatrics.aappublications.org/content/pediatrics/122/Supplement_2/S69.full.pdf.

34. Taddio, Anna, Rebecca Pillai Riddell, Moshe Ipp, Steven Moss, Stephen Baker, Jonathan Tolkin, Dave Malini, Sharmeen Feerasta, Preeya Govan, Emma Fletcher, Horace Wong, Caitlin McNair, Priyanjali Mithal, and Derek Stephens. "Relative Effectiveness of Additive Pain Interventions during Vaccination in Infants." *Canadian Medical Association Journal* 189, no. 6 (December 2016): 1–9. P. 8. http://www.cmaj.ca/content/early/2016/12/12/cmaj.160542.full.pdf+html.

35. Wisner, Katherine L., Dorothy K. Y. Sit, Mary C. McShea, David M. Rizzo, Rebecca A. Zoretich, Carolyn L. Hughes, Heather F. Eng, James F. Luther, Stephen R. Wisniewski, Michelle L. Costantino, Andrea L. Confer, Eydie L. Moses-Kolko, Christopher S. Famy, and Barbara H. Hanusa. "Onset Timing, Thoughts of Self-Harm, and Diagnoses in Postpartum Women with Screen-Positive Depression Findings." *JAMA Psychiatry*, published online March 13, 2013: E1–E9. https://adaa.org/sites/default/files/Barnes184-2.pdf.

36. "Baby Blues: Causes, Symptoms and Treatment." American Pregnancy Association, May 18, 2016. Accessed July 03, 2017. http://americanpregnancy.org/first-year-of-life/baby-blues/.

37. Ibid.

38. "Do I Have a Form of Postpartum Depression?" American Pregnancy Association, May 18, 2016. Accessed July 03, 2017. http://americanpregnancy.org/first-year-of-life/forms-of-postpartum-depression/.

39. "Postpartum Depression Facts." National Institute of Mental Health. Accessed July 3, 2017. https://www.nimh.nih.gov/health/publications/postpartum-depression-facts/index.shtml.

40. American Pregnancy Association, "Do I Have a Form of Postpartum Depression?"

41. Ibid.

42. Ibid.

43. Ellis, Jessica. "Shocking Stats Reveal That Nine out of Ten Mums Feel Pressure to Be 'Perfect.' Who Is to Blame for This?" HuffPost UK Parent Voices, April 5, 2017. http://www.huffingtonpost.co.uk/jessica-ellis/shocking-stats-reveal-tha_b_15813968.html.

44. Hanson, Rick, Jan Hanson, and Ricki Pollycove. *Mother Nurture: A Mother's Guide to Health in Body, Mind, and Intimate Relationships.* New York: Penguin Books, 2002. P. 12.

45. Mejia, Robin. "Green Exercise May Be Good for Your Head." *Environmental Science and Technology* 44, no. 10 (2010): 3649. http://pubs.acs.org/doi/full/10.1021/es101129n.

46. "Women's, Men's Brains Respond Differently to Hungry Infant's Cries." National Institutes of Health, May 6, 2013. Accessed July 23, 2017. https://www.nih.gov/news-events/news-releases/womens-mens-brains-respond-differently-hungry-infants-cries.

47. Dunstan, Priscilla. *Calm the Crying: The Secret Baby Language That Reveals the Hidden Meaning behind an Infant's Cry.* New York: Avery, 2012. Pp. 29, 33, 36, 103, 107.

48. Karp, Harvey. *The Happiest Baby on the Block: The New Way to Calm Crying and Help Your Newborn Baby Sleep Longer,* Second Edition. New York: Bantam Books, 2015. P. 129.

49. Sears, William, and Martha Sears. *The Attachment Parenting Book: A Commonsense Guide to Understanding and Nurturing Your Baby.* Boston: Little, Brown, 2001. P. 27.

50. Partanen, Eino, Teija Kujala, Mari Tervaniemi, and Minna Huotilainen. "Prenatal Music Exposure Induces Long-Term Neural Effects." *PLoS ONE* 8, no. 10 (2013): e78946. https://doi.org/10.1371/journal.pone.0078946.

51. Moore, Elizabeth R., Gene C. Anderson, Nils Bergman, and Therese Dowswell. "Early Skin-to-Skin Contact for Mothers and Their Healthy Newborn Infants." *Cochrane Database of Systematic Reviews* 5 (2012): CD003519. Accessed July 5, 2017. https://www.ncbi.nlm.nih.gov/pmc/articles/PMC3979156/.

52. Borreli, Lizette. "Your Baby's Crying in Sleep Could Lead You to Lose 44 Days of Slumber in a Single Year." Medical Daily, September 18, 2013. http://www.medicaldaily.com/your-babys-crying-sleep-could-lead-you-lose-44-days-slumber-single-year-257149.

53. "How Much Sleep Do We Really Need?" National Sleep Foundation: Excessive Sleepiness. Accessed July 25, 2017. https://sleepfoundation.org/excessivesleepiness/content/how-much-sleep-do-we-really-need-0.

54. Ding, Karisa. "Sleep Deprivation and New Parents." Health Day, last updated January 20, 2017. Accessed August 14, 2017. https://consumer.healthday.com/encyclopedia/parenting-31/parenting-health-news-525/sleep-deprivation-and-new-parents-643886.html.

55. Mindell, Jodi A. *Sleeping Through the Night: How Infants, Toddlers, and Their Parents Can Get a Good Night's Sleep.* New York: HarperCollins, 2005. P. 297.

56. "The Ideal Temperature for Sleep." Sleep.Org, powered by the National Sleep Foundation. https://sleep.org/articles/temperature-for-sleep/.

57. Pantley, Elizabeth. *The No-Cry Sleep Solution: Gentle Ways to Help Your Baby Sleep Through the Night.* New York: McGraw-Hill, 2002. P. 69.

58. Mindell, Jodi A., Erin S. Leichman, Courtney DuMond, and Avi Sadeh. "Sleep and Social-Emotional Development in Infants and Toddlers." *Journal of Clinical Child & Adolescent Psychology*, 46, no. 2 (Mar–Apr 2017): 236–46.

59. Mindell, *Sleeping Through the Night*, p. 75.

60. Ibid., 100–1.

61. Ibid., 139.

62. "American Academy of Pediatrics Announces New Safe Sleep Recommendations to Protect Against SIDS, Sleep-Related Infant Deaths." American Academy of Pediatrics. https://www.aap.org/en-us/about-the-aap/aap-press-room/pages/american-academy-of-pediatrics-announces-new-safe-sleep-recommendations-to-protect-against-sids.aspx.

63. Ibid.

64. Sears, Martha, and William Sears. *The Breastfeeding Book: Everything You Need to Know About Nursing Your Child from Birth Through Weaning*. Boston, MA: Little, Brown, 2000. P. 53.

65. Murkoff, Heidi, and Sharon Mazel. *What to Expect the First Year*, Third Edition. Sydney: HarperCollins, 2015. P. 417.

66. Shapiro, Alyson Fearnley, John M. Gottman, and Sybil Carrère. "The Baby and the Marriage: Identifying Factors That Buffer Against Decline in Marital Satisfaction After the First Baby Arrives." *Journal of Family Psychology* 14, no. 1 (2000): 59–70. http://webspace.pugetsound.edu/facultypages/cjones/adoldev/Shapiro-Bringing%20Baby%20Home.pdf.

67. Hirschberger, Gilad, Sanjay Srivastava, Penny Marsh, Carolyn Pape Cowan, and Philip A. Cowan. "Attachment, Marital Satisfaction, and Divorce During the First Fifteen Years of Parenthood." *Personal Relationships* 16, no. 3 (September 2009): 401–20. https://www.ncbi.nlm.nih.gov/pmc/articles/PMC3061469/.

68. Shapiro, "The Baby and the Marriage," p. 60.

69. National Poll on Children's Health. "Mom Shaming or Constructive Criticism? Perspectives of Mothers." *Mott Poll Report* 29, no. 3 (June 19, 2017). Accessed July 10, 2017. http://mottnpch.org/reports-surveys/mom-shaming-or-constructive-criticism-perspectives-mothers.

70. The American Academy of Pediatrics Task Force on Sudden Infant Death Syndrome. "SIDS and Other Sleep-Related Infant Deaths: Expansion of Recommendations for a Safe Infant Sleeping Environment." *Pediatrics* 128, no. 5 (2011): e1341–67. Accessed July 10, 2017. http://pediatrics.aappublications.org/content/pediatrics/128/5/e1341.full.pdf.

71. Sears, William. "The Effects of Excessive Crying." *Ask Dr. Sears*, May 17, 2016. Accessed July 10, 2017. http://www.askdrsears.com/topics/health-concerns/fussy-baby/science-says-excessive-crying-could-be-harmful.

ABOUT THE AUTHOR

MARIA LIANOS-CARBONE is a mom of two, social media strategist, and publisher of amotherworld.com, a leading lifestyle blog for women who happen to be moms. Life doesn't stop after kids!

Also a freelance writer, Maria's work has been published in *Huffington Post Canada*, Babble.com, *Canadian Living*, *Today's Parent*, and *Parents Canada*. Maria has worked on digital campaigns with brands such as Rogers, Air Canada, American Express, P&G, Costco, TD Canada Trust, Walmart, and more. She has appeared as a guest on *CNN Newsroom*, CBC's *Marketplace*, *The Mom Show*, and *Rogers Daytime*.

ABOUT FAMILIUS

Visit Our Website: www.familius.com

Join Our Family

There are lots of ways to connect with us! Subscribe to our newsletters at www.familius.com to receive uplifting daily inspiration, essays from our Pater Familius, a free ebook every month, and the first word on special discounts and Familius news.

Get Bulk Discounts

If you feel a few friends and family might benefit from what you've read, let us know and we'll be happy to provide you with quantity discounts. Simply email us at orders@familius.com.

Connect

- Facebook: www.facebook.com/paterfamilius
- Twitter: @familiustalk, @paterfamilius1
- Pinterest: www.pinterest.com/familius
- Instagram: @familiustalk

FAMILIUS

The most important work you ever do will be within the walls of your own home.

CPSIA information can be obtained
at www.ICGtesting.com
Printed in the USA
LVOW03s2337080218
565866LV00003B/7/P